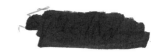

Magnet Therapy

An Alternative Medicine Definitive Guide

by WILLIAM H. PHILPOTT, M.D., *and* DWIGHT K. KALITA, PH.D.,

with BURTON GOLDBERG

ALTERNATIVEMEDICINE.COM BOOKS
TIBURON, CALIFORNIA

AlternativeMedicine.com, Inc.
1640 Tiburon Blvd., Suite 2
Tiburon, CA 94920
www.alternativemedicine.com

Art Director: Janine White
Production Manager: Gail Gongoll
Production Assistance: Victoria Swart
Cover Design: Anne Walzer

Manufactured in the United States of America.

10 9 8 7 6 5 4 3 2

Library of Congress Cataloging-in-Publication Data

Philpott, William H., 1919-
    Magnet therapy: an alternative medicine definitive guide / by William H.
Philpott and Dwight K. Kalita with Burton Goldberg.
        p. cm.
    Includes bibliographical references and index.
    ISBN 1-887299-21-1 (pbk.)
    1. Magnetotherapy. I. Kalita, Dwight K. II. Goldberg, Burton, 1926- III. Title.

RM893.P47 2000
618.8'45—dc21   00-044176
                    CIP

Contents

PART ONE
Magnet Basics

PART TWO
An A-Z of Health Conditions with Magnet Therapy Success Stories

About the Authors

William H. Philpott, M.D., has specialty training and practice in psychiatry, electroencephalography, neurology, nutrition, environmental medicine, and toxicology. He is a fellow of the Society of Environmental Medicine and Toxicology and also the Orthomolecular Psychiatric Society. He is a founding member of the Academy of Orthomolecular Psychiatry. His research into the causes of major mental illnesses and degenerative diseases resulted in the publication of the books *Brain Allergies and Victory Over Diabetes*.

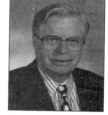

After 40 years of medical practice, Dr. Philpott retired in 1990 to engage in research as Chairman of the Independent Institutional Review Board. In this capacity, he guides physicians gathering data on the treatment and prevention of degenerative diseases using magnetic therapy.

Dwight K. Kalita, Ph.D., is the co-author of *Brain Allergies, Victory Over Diabetes*, and *Nourishing Your Child*, and the author of *Light Consciousness*. He was also co-editor of *A Physician's Handbook on Orthomolecular Medicine*. He has devoted over 30 years to medical journalism and to the position of Research Director of the Bio-Ecologic Research Center in Ohio. Dr. Kalita has published frequently for general interest and professional publications.

User's Guide

One of the features of this book is that it is interactive, thanks to the following icons:

This means you can turn to the listed pages elsewhere in this book for more information.

Many times the text mentions a medical term that requires explanation. We don't want to interrupt the text, so instead we put the explanation in the margins under this icon.

This tells you where to contact a physician, group, or publication mentioned in the text. This is an editorial service to our readers. All items are based on recommendations from the clinical practice of physicians in this book. The publisher has no financial interest in any clinic, physician, or product discussed in this book.

This sign tells you there may be some risks, uncertainties, side effects, or special contraindications regarding a procedure or substance.

Here we refer you to our best-selling book, *Alternative Medicine: The Definitive Guide*, for more information on a particular topic.

Here we refer you to our book *Alternative Medicine Definitive Guide to Cancer* for more information on a particular topic.

Here we refer you to our book *Alternative Medicine Definitive Guide to Headaches* for more information on a particular topic.

Here we refer you to our book *The Enzyme Cure* for more information on enzymes and how they can be used to relieve health problems.

Here we refer you to our book *The Supplement Shopper* for more information on nutritional supplements for various health conditions.

Here we refer you to our book *Weight Loss: An Alternative Medicine Definitive Guide* for more information on a particular topic.

Here we refer you to our book *Cancer Diagnosis: What To Do Next* for more information on a particular topic.

Important Information

Burton Goldberg and the editors of *Alternative Medicine* are proud of the public and professional praise accorded AlternativeMedicine.com's (formerly Future Medicine Publishing) series of books. This latest book in the series continues the groundbreaking tradition of its predecessors.

Your health and that of your loved ones is important. Treat this book as an educational tool which will enable you to better understand, assess, and choose the best course of treatment when health problems arise, and how to prevent health problems from developing in the first place.

Remember that this book is different. This book is about alternative approaches to health—approaches generally not understood and, at this time, not endorsed by the medical establishment. We urge you to discuss the treatments described in this book with your doctor. If your doctor is open-minded, you may actually educate him or her. We have been gratified to learn that many of our readers have found their physicians open to the new ideas presented to them.

Use this book wisely. As many of the treatments described in this book are, by definition, alternative, they have not been investigated, approved, or endorsed by any government or regulatory agency. National, state, and local laws may vary regarding the use and application of many of the treatments discussed. The authors and publisher of this book do not claim that magnets will cure any degenerative disease. Accordingly, this book should not be substituted for the advice and care of a physician or other licensed health-care professional. Pregnant women, in particular, are urged to consult a physician before commencing any therapy. Ultimately, you must take responsibility for your health and how you use the information in this book.

AlternativeMedicine.com and the authors have no financial interest in any of the products or services discussed in this book, with one exception. The book makes references to AlternativeMedicine.com's other publications. All of the factual information in this book has been drawn from the scientific literature. To protect privacy, all patient names have been changed. Branded products and services discussed in the book are evaluated solely on the independent and direct experience of the health-care practitioners quoted. Reference to them does not imply an endorsement nor a superiority over other branded products and services which may provide similar or superior results.

You Don't Have to Suffer with Ill Health

HEALTH PROBLEMS are not something you have to live with—alternative medicine has practical solutions for identifying and treating the underlying causes and can bring lasting relief for a myriad of diseases. Many people have learned this the hard way, living with discomfort and pain for years before discovering that there is another option. Alternative medicine recognizes that illnesses do not have one cause, but multiple factors that together overload your body systems. Looking at illness and health in this way makes for more effective treatment than the single-cause focus of conventional medicine. In this book, you will learn that once you identify the hidden factors that are combining to produce your illness, you can treat each one using magnet therapy and permanently eliminate your symptoms. Patient success stories throughout the book provide practical details on how others were able to reverse their health problems using magnet therapy.

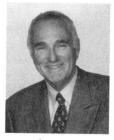

Conventional medicine generally offers drug treatments that may temporarily relieve your symptoms, but also introduce serious side effects. Alternative medicine physicians, on the other hand, focus on finding the root causes, rather than merely trying to alleviate symptoms. In this book, we show you how to treat a number of illnesses using safe, noninvasive magnet therapy. Two primary conditions in the body set the groundwork for illness—high acidity and a lack of oxygen. Magnet therapy, by normalizing these factors and producing a number of other health-promoting effects, prevents and reverses ill health.

Alternative medicine looks at the whole person, considering the individual's symptoms, health history, diet, and underlying imbalances. Healing these underlying causes leading to illness brings lasting relief, not a simple masking of symptoms. This is the basic principle of alternative medicine and the reason why it succeeds where conventional medicine often fails in treatment of chronic disease.

This book is here to tell you that you don't have to live with ill-

This book is here to tell you that you don't have to live with illness, or with a continuing cycle of drugs and their side effects. By treating what is actually causing the condition, not only can health problems be reversed using magnet therapy, but your overall health will be improved.

ness, or with a continuing cycle of drugs and their side effects. By treating what is actually causing the condition, not only can health problems be reversed using magnet therapy, but your overall health will be improved. Start with the therapies in this book to relieve your symptoms and eliminate your illness for good. God bless.

—Burton Goldberg

Visit our website at
www.alternativemedicine.com

Part One

Magnet Basics

1

What is Magnet Therapy?

ELECTROMAGNETIC ENERGY is an integral part of the human body. It can help produce illness and help bring healing, depending on its type and strength. The world is surrounded by magnetic fields: some are generated by the Earth's magnetism, others by solar storms and changes in the weather. Magnetic fields are also created by everyday electrical devices: motors, televisions, office equipment, computers, electrically heated water beds, electric blankets, microwave ovens, the electrical wiring in homes, and the power lines that supply them.

Recently, scientists have discovered that external magnetic fields can affect the body's functioning in both positive and negative ways, and this observation has led to the development of magnetic field therapy. The use of magnets and electrical devices to generate controlled magnetic fields has many medical applications and has proven to be one of the most effective means available for diagnosing human illness.

Magnets and electromagnetic therapy devices are now being used to relieve symptoms and reverse degenerative diseases, eliminate pain, facilitate the healing of broken bones, counter the effects of stress, and address the reversal of cancer. Magnets are widely used throughout Europe and are now becoming more accepted in the United States. Researchers have noted that positive and negative magnetic energies have different effects upon the biological systems of animals and humans—negative magnetic fields have a beneficial effect, whereas positive magnetic fields have a stressful effect. They have found that magnets could be used in the treatment of arthritis, cancer, glaucoma, infertility, mental and emotional disorders, and other diseases.

The Basics of Magnetic Fields

Magnetic fields are everywhere, originating from the Earth, the weather, and the numerous electrical devices in our lives. Even the human body produces subtle magnetic fields, generated by chemical reactions within cells and in the nervous system.[1]

Almost anything can be magnetized—it's not just a property of iron and other metals. Magnetism happens on an atomic level, where tiny charged particles called electrons orbit around the atom like planets around the sun. These electrons also spin, like the earth on its axis, creating miniature magnetic fields with a north and a south pole. If you can get all of these electrons spinning in the same direction, you get magnetism.[2]

So, magnetism is an alignment of electrons in iron or other materials in a uniform direction between opposite magnetic poles, forming a balance of positive and negative fields. Magnetic fields affect other matter, for example, attracting or repelling the electrons in other objects. That is how you tell if a magnetic field is present: the effect of magnetic force on objects in that field. The power of the magnetic field gets stronger as more electrons become aligned.[3] The most common source of magnetic fields is electric currents. Magnetism is a product of the flow of electrons in a direct current (DC) circuit. With suitable materials, a DC circuit produces a permanent static field magnet.

The term *electromagnetic* is used synonymously for *magnetic* or *magnetism* and these terms will be used interchangeably in this book. The term *magnetism* often has a pejorative ring to it (associated with mesmerism or "animal magnetism") when used by those who would seek to discredit the use of magnets as a medical therapy.[4]

The Spin on Magnetic Fields

A static magnetic field is an energy field by virtue of the movement of electrons in that field.[5] Magnetic fields provide two types of energy response: the negative field spins electrons counterclockwise and the positive field spins electrons clockwise. The spinning of electrons in negative and positive fields is opposite and the biological responses to these magnetic fields are also opposite.[6] Technically speaking, magnetic fields are three-dimensional, so the electrons actually spiral-spin.

A magnet is an object surrounded by a magnetic field that can attract iron or steel. All magnets have two poles: one is called a north pole (negative) and the other a south pole (positive). Opposite poles, like north and south, attract whereas like poles (north and north or south and south) repel.[7] A direct current electric circuit can serve to line up specific metals and produce the static magnetic field of a permanent magnet. All matter has some magnetic properties, but permanent magnets commonly contain one or two magnetizable metals: iron oxide and the rare earth metal neodymium. That is because the atoms in these materials align to a magnetic field more strongly.[8] Once aligned, these magnetizable metals are held firmly in a hard substance, such as ceramic or plastic.

Naming Magnetic Poles—The poles of a magnet can be determined with a magnetometer. This instrument is composed of a compass that registers the presence of positive and negative electromagnetic poles (to locate the poles, the arrowhead of the needle marked "N" or "North" will point to the magnet's negative pole). A magnetometer can also determine the positive and negative poles of an electric current. Throughout this book, magnetic fields are described as positive and negative, based on the electric definition of electromagnetism formed by a DC circuit. A magnetometer converts the geographic description of polarity to the electromagnetic definition. This use of *positive* and *negative* as applied to magnetism is recommended rather than the geographic definitions, which may cause confusion in regard to human physiology.

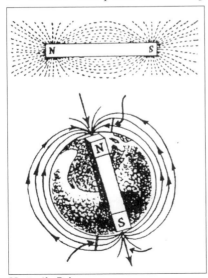

Magnetic Poles.

Magnet Strength—The strength of a magnet is measured in units of gauss, named after Carl Friedrich Gauss, a 19th-century German mathematician and physicist. One gauss is equivalent to about twice the average strength of the earth's magnetic field. The Tesla is another common magnetic measurement, named after Nikola Tesla, a Serbian-American who did extensive research in electromagnetism. One Tesla equals 10,000 gauss.

Magnetic devices mentioned in this book have a manufacturer's gauss rating to inform you of the magnet's strength. However, the actual strength of the magnet at the skin surface is often much less than this number. For example, a 4,000-gauss magnet transmits about 1,200 gauss therapeutically and magnets placed in pillows or bed pads will render even lower amounts of field strength, because a magnet's strength quickly decreases with the distance from the subject. The overall size and thickness of a magnet affects the depth of penetration.

Magnetic Fields are Vital to Health

The human body produces subtle magnetic fields that are generated by the chemical reactions within the cells and the ionic currents of the nervous system.[9] Neurons are electromagnetic positive and their axons (the branch of the neuron that conducts nerve impulses away) are electromagnetic negative, so that the nervous system functions on a direct current basis. Recently, scientists have discovered that external magnetic fields can also affect the body's functioning in both positive and negative ways, and this observation has led to the development of magnetic field therapy.

Humans need both internal and external sources of magnetic fields for survival. Internally, the human body makes mineral (magnetite) crystals that can be magnetized. These magnetized crystals, containing iron and manganese, are found in the pineal gland (located in the center of the brain), ethmoid magnetic organ (a bone forming the nasal cavity), and neurons. These organs and structures in the body are actually permanent static field magnets that generate magnetic fields. Individual cells have paramagnetic fields centered in the DNA, produced by the biochemical processing of nutrients, water, and oxygen.

An external magnetic field can also magnetize the crystals produced in the body. Physiologists agree that humans receive approximately 30% of their energy from external sources.[10] The body also

Electromagnetic Fields Can Be Detrimental to Your Health

According to Robert Becker, M.D., John Zimmerman, Ph.D., and many other scientists and researchers, we live in an environment that is filled with stress-producing, electromagnetic fields generated by the electrical wiring in homes and offices, as well as from televisions, computers, microwave ovens, over-head lights, electrical poles, and the hundreds of motors that can generate higher than naturally occurring gauss strengths.

The frequency at which a magnetic field is pulsed determines whether or not it is harmful. For example, the voltage of the electrical current used in homes in the United States is 60 cycles per second. In contrast, normal frequencies of the human brain during waking hours range from eight to 22 cycles per second, while in sleep the frequencies may drop to as low as two cycles per second. The higher frequencies present in electrical currents may disturb the brain's natural resonant frequencies and, in time, lead to cellular fatigue, according to Dr. Zimmerman.

In 1979, Nancy Wertheimer, Ph.D., an epidemiologist at the University of Colorado, found that there was a statistically significant increase in childhood cancers among those who were exposed to the AC (alternating current) electromagnetic fields, which emanate from the electrical power lines that run along many of the nation's city streets.[13] Ten years later, a large-scale study conducted by the New York State Department of Health confirmed Dr. Wertheimer's findings and added that it also affected the neuro-hormones of the brain.[14] In 1988, Marjorie Speers, Ph.D., at the University of Texas Medical Branch, found that workers exposed to electro-magnetic fields showed a 13-fold increase in brain tumors compared to the unexposed group.[15] Other studies have shown increases in suicides,[16] depression,[17] chromosomal abnormalities,[18] and learning difficulties.[19]

In another study by Dr. Wertheimer, it was observed that users of electric blankets had a higher incidence of miscarriages.[20] Add to this the possible perils from fluorescent lighting, microwave ovens, hair dryers, electric shavers, and heaters, and one can see why more research is urgently needed. "Only a few farsighted individuals, such as Dr. Becker, have given much thought to the fact that the new electromagnetic environment created by 20th-century technology may be exerting subtle, yet very important, effects upon biology," states Dr. Zimmerman. "This may include alterations in gene expression, immune function, viral pathogenesis, and future genetic tendencies."

absorbs electromagnetic energy from the environment through oxygen and water, which are paramagnetic (capable of being magnetized).[11] Also, blood flowing in the body is flowing through the

Earth's magnetic field, which produces electro-motive energy. These sources of magnetic fields can influence body function. A negative magnet-ic field can favorably affect cell function, pH level (acidity or alkalinity), hormone production, enzyme activity, energy production from ATP (SEE QUICK DEFINITION), healing, and growth. Thus, negative magnetic fields can serve as sys-temic defenses against disease.

Many people are becoming aware that our external sources of magnetism are currently dwindling. Kyoichi Nakagawa, M.D., references authorities who have demonstrated that the Earth's magnetic field has diminished in half over the last 500 years. Nakagawa points out that modern technology, such as trains, cars, and metal buildings, absorb the Earth's magnetic field and cause a loss of gauss strength. This interferes with the human energy system because electromagnetic induction does not occur at an optimum level. It seems logical that the human body is adapted to a higher gauss strength than that of the Earth's current magnetic field, and thus human deficiencies are now emerging.

After more than 20 years of research, Nakagawa has concluded that a magnetic field deficiency syndrome exists as a result of this weakened magnetism. The symptoms of this syndrome include: stiffness in the shoulders, back, and neck; chest pains; headache and heaviness of the head; dizziness; insom-nia; habitual constipation; and general lassitude.[12] The long-term biological consequences of magnetic deficiency include the follow-ing: the development of acute symptoms and chronic degenerative diseases; the loss of normal healing ability; and the unsuccessful defense against infectious microorganisms and environmental tox-ins. In particular, when the body's supply of magnetism is deficient, the oxidoreductase enzymes do not function properly. These enzymes are needed for the following: the reversal of free radicals (SEE QUICK DEFINITION), hydrogen peroxide, aldehydes, alcohols, and acids back to molecular oxygen; and the maintenance of the pH at a normal alkaline state. A negative magnetic field activates paramagnetic bicarbonates in the body and activates these enzymes.

QUICK DEFINITION

ATP stands for adenosine triphosphate, a substance found in all cells, particularly muscle, and responsible for energy. When enzymes split ATP, energy is released from the high-energy phosphate bonds. This bond can be instantly split on demand whenever energy is required to run cellular functions. ATP is often called the cell's energy currency because it can be continually spent and remade again in a mat-ter of minutes.

For more on the **physiological effects of magnets**, see Chapter 2: How Magnets Heal, pp. 26-36.

Magnets as a Medical Therapy

For more about **magnet therapy for mental Illness**, see Mental Illness.

Electromagnetic energy and the human body have a valid and important interrelationship. Magnetic field therapy can be used in both diagnosing and treating physical and emotional disorders. This process has been recognized to relieve symptoms and may, in some cases, retard the cycle of new disease. Magnets and electromagnetic therapy devices are now being used to relieve symptoms and reverse degenerative diseases, ease pain, speed the healing of broken bones, and counter the effects of stress.

The use of magnets and electrical devices to generate controlled magnetic fields has proven to be one of the most effective means for diagnosing disease. For example, MRI (magnetic resonance imaging) is replacing X-ray diagnosis because it is safer and more accurate, and magnetoencephalography is now replacing electroencephalography (EEG) as the preferred technique for recording the brain's electrical activity.

In 1974, physicist Albert Roy Davis noted that positive and negative magnetic polarities have different effects upon biological systems. He found that magnets could be used to kill cancer cells in animals, and could also be used in the treatment of arthritis, infertility, and chronic diseases related to aging.[21] He concluded that negative magnetic fields have a beneficial effect on living organisms, whereas positive magnetic fields are detrimental (stressful).

The negative pole calms neurons and encourages rest, relaxation, and sleep. When sufficiently high in gauss strength, it can even produce general anesthesia. And because it is neuron-calming, it has been successfully used in the control of neurosis, psychosis, seizures, addictive withdrawal, and movement disorders. A negative magnetic field consistently produces a predictable, long-term healing response, because only this field can ultimately relieve stress or injury. The body itself always responds with negative magnetic field energy to counter any stressor. The negative magnetic field counteracts stress by the following mechanisms: normalization of pH (acid-base balance), correction of cellular swelling or edema, and release of molecular oxygen.

In contrast, the positive pole has a stressful effect on the body. With a prolonged exposure, it interferes with metabolic functioning, produces acidity, reduces cellular oxygen, and encourages the spread of latent microorganisms. As a neurologist, I have seen that a positive magnetic field excites or stimulates neurons. The higher the gauss strength of the positive pole, the higher the level of stimulation. In fact, a sufficiently high positive magnetic field can even evoke seizures and precipitate psychosis in those so predisposed.

"Scientifically designed, double-blind, placebo-controlled studies, however, have not been done to substantiate the claims of there being different effects between positive and negative magnetic poles," says John Zimmerman, Ph.D., President of the Bio-Electro-Magnetics Institute. "But numerous anecdotal, clinical observations suggest that such differences are real and do exist. Clearly, scientific research is needed to substantiate these claims."

A Brief History of Magnet Therapy

While magnet therapy may just now be gaining more widespread use and popularity in the United States and elsewhere, the use of magnetic energy for healing dates back thousands of years. In fact, the earliest written medical text, *The Yellow Emperor's Book of Internal Medicine*, published in China around 2,000 B.C., mentions the application of 'magnetic stones" to correct health imbalances.[22]

The ancient Egyptians were apparently acquainted with the power of magnets. Legend has it that Cleopatra slept with a magnetic stone on her forehead to preserve her youthful appearance (perhaps trying to cause the pineal gland in the brain to release melatonin). The ancient Hindus in India believed that a dying person should rest with their body aligned north and south (their head pointed north) to relieve their pain and ease their departure from this life.[23]

The word *magnet* comes from the ancient Greeks. It is thought to derive from *Magnes lithos*, meaning "stone from Magnesia," an area of Greece that was known for its volcanic rocks with magnetic attributes. The Greek philosopher Aristotle spoke about using magnets as a healing therapy.

The next promulgator of magnet therapy was Paracelsus, a physician and alchemist born in Switzerland in 1493. He was the first to propose that illnesses were caused by external substances (the concept of disease), not imbalances in the body's "humors" (the dominant theory at the time). He recommended using sulfur, mercury, and other substances to treat diseases. Paracelsus had a notion of a "life force" in nature and the human body, which he called *archaeus* (meaning "ancient"). He treated illnesses by replenishing the archaeus with the energy found in certain herbs and foods. Paracelsus advocated using magnets to energize and influence the body's life force to start the healing process, treating everything from inflammation to diarrhea to epilepsy.[24]

In 1600, William Gilbert, court physician to Elizabeth I of England, published the first scientific treatise on magnetism, *De Magnete*. This book summarized the current knowledge about magnetism, showing, for instance, that steel holds a magnetic charge better than iron and that there is a distinction between magnetism and electricity. Gilbert was the first to describe the Earth as a huge magnet with magnetic poles close to the geographic north and south poles. He also confirmed that use of the lodestone could be "beneficial in many diseases of the human system."[25] (The term *lodestone* for magnetized stones is from the Middle Ages, when the lodestone—"guiding stone"—was used in compasses by sailors as a navigational tool.)[26]

Franz Anton Mesmer, an 18th-century mathematician and physician, wrote his doctoral thesis on the effects of gravitational fields on human health. He proposed that there was magnetic energy flowing throughout the universe and inside the body as well. Mesmer thought that the body had magnetic poles and that illness was caused by these poles moving out of alignment with the universal magnetic flow. He experimented with using magnets to treat seizures and other conditions.

Mesmer claimed that he could heal by touch, applying his own magnetism to influence the magnetic flow in a patient's body. Mesmer believed that magnetism could treat mental illnesses directly and other conditions indirectly. He became famous traveling around Europe as a healer and he later opened a magnetism salon in Paris. In his salon, patients sat in water-filled vats containing iron filings and rods. Patients would pour magnetic water on parts of their bodies affected by illness and sometimes join hands to facilitate the magnetic flow, all accompanied by music and colored lights added by the theatrical Mesmer. Patients sometimes fainted or went into convulsions, later claiming they were "mesmerized." (Mesmer's notion of magnetism gradually came to be viewed as hypnotic suggestion, hence the current meaning of the word *mesmerize*.)[27]

Around 1800, Alessandro Volta constructed the first battery (made of silver, moist cardboard, and zinc), which produced a small, steady electric current. Further experiments with electricity by Andre-Marie Ampere, Michael Faraday, and others, established the link between magnetism and electricity. Faraday demonstrated that a magnet in motion could produce electricity and that the flow of electricity produces a magnetic field. This was confirmed by Scottish scientist James Maxwell, who showed that light was an electromagnetic phenomenon as well.

The publication of Mary Shelley's *Frankenstein* in 1818 certainly shows that electricity was in the air during this period. This gothic romance about bringing the dead to life reflected an interest at this time in using electromagnetism as a therapy. Reanimation devices, using electricity in much the same way as defibrillators are used in hospitals today to jumpstart the heart, became popular and were successfully used for heart arrhythmias, angina, and curvature of the spine. Magnetic boots, rings, girdles, and caps, as well as magnetic ointments were available in mail-order catalogues. Daniel Palmer founded Palmer's School of Magnetic Cure in Davenport, Iowa, which taught massage techniques, spinal manipulations, and magnets as healing therapies—this later evolved into modern chiropractic.[28]

The discovery of the electron at the end of the 19th century moved electromagnetism to the atomic level, demonstrating that all matter is essentially electric in nature. Finally, Albert Einstein, in postulating his general theory of relativity, showed that electricity and magnetism are not discrete phenomena, but different aspects of the same phenomenon.[29] Medical textbooks at this time included magnetism and electricity as therapeutic alternatives for mental disorders in particular and other conditions as well. It was recommended for convulsions, insomnia, migraine, fatigue, arthritis, and pain. Magnet therapy fell into disfavor following World War II with the development of antiobiotics and biochemistry-based medicine. Today, magnet therapy is seeing a resurgence in use and is an officially approved therapy in over 45 countries worldwide.[30]

The Future of Magnet Therapy

With the rising popularity of magnetic field diagnostic techniques such as MRI (magnetic resonance imaging), magnets and electromagnetic devices are beginning to gain mainstream medical acceptance as diagnostic and treatment tools. Eventually, the medical

Magnetic therapy in the future will be seen not only as a valuable diagnostic technique, but as an effective treatment modality. Because magnets do not introduce any foreign substance to the body, this makes them safer over the long-term than medications.

For more about **magnet therapy for arteriosclerosis and other forms of heart disease**, see Heart Disease.

community will understand that magnetic therapy as a treatment modality provides predictable and effective results for a variety of illnesses. Magnetic therapy in the future will be seen not only as a valuable diagnostic technique, but as an effective treatment modality. Because magnets do not introduce any foreign substance to the body, this makes them safer over the long-term than medications.

As our understanding of magnetic energy improves, we will begin to see that the negative magnetic field produces the most effective relief of pain caused by infections, local edema, acidosis, and toxicity. Magnets will also prove central to the healing process, particularly with broken bones, bruises, burns, acute environmental allergies, and chronic degenerative diseases.

Negative magnetic field therapy will be a major tool in relieving arteriosclerosis (hardening of the arteries), Alzheimer's, high cholesterol, and high triglycerides. It will resolve problems related to calcium metabolism, including some types of kidney stones as well as insoluble calcium deposits around joints and in the brain. All types of cancer will prove reversible by continuous exposure to a negative magnetic field. Negative magnetic field therapy will prove effective in reverting scar tissue to normal tissue.

Negative magnetic field therapy will be the most effectual antibiotic treatment for infections (bacteria, viruses, fungi, and parasites). Indeed, a negative magnetic field will become the antibiotic of tomorrow, because none of these organisms can tolerate a negative magnetic field. This antibiotic effect will be of tremendous value because conventional medicine is currently having difficulties making new antibiotics fast enough to counter microorganism mutations, which render antibiotics ineffective.

For more about **magnet therapy and infections**, see Infections. For more about **magnet therapy and mental illness**, see Mental Illness.

Negative magnetic field therapy will offer the greatest control over abnormal electromagnetic activity in the central nervous system. Negative magnetic exposure will be used to control major mental disorders (delusions, hallucinations, disassociation, obsessive-compulsiveness, psychotic depression, and others) as well as minor emotional disorders (all types of neuroses) and learning and behavioral disorders (dyslexia, attention deficit disorder, hyperactivity). Negative magnetic field therapy will be shown to be an effective stimulator of the health-enhancing hormones melatonin and human growth hormone (HGH) when used at night. This application of magnets can sub-stantially replace tranquilizers, antidepressants, and anti-seizure medications in the treatment of mental illness. In addition, it will help correct sleep disorders.

CHAPTER

2

How Magnets Heal

ANEGATIVE MAGNETIC FIELD produces a number of healthful reactions in the body that can help eliminate the symptoms and causes of chronic illnesses. The body itself produces a negative magnetic field to speed healing, but if your system is compromised by poor nutrition or lifestyle choices, your body may not be able to heal itself. Applying an external source of magnetic energy can boost your recuperative powers.

"Magnetic field therapy is a method that penetrates the whole human body and can treat every organ without chemical side effects," according to Wolfgang Ludwig, Sc.D., Ph.D., Director of the Institute for Biophysics in Horb, Germany. Magnetic field therapy has been used effectively in the treatment of many conditions, including cancer, rheumatoid diseases, infections and inflammation, headaches (including migraines), insomnia and other sleep disorders, circulatory problems, fractures and pain, and environmental illness. Dr. Ludwig adds that magnetic changes in the environment can affect the electromagnetic balance of the human organism and contribute to disease. Magnetic therapy can be used to counter the effects caused by the electromagnetic pollution in the environment.

Such a treatment program can last from just a few minutes to overnight, depending upon the situation and severity. It can also involve magnets being applied to our bodies several times a day or for even days or weeks at a time.

The results of magnetic therapy can be quite dramatic. For example, Stan, 46, had suffered for years from severe heart flutter, diarrhea, and nausea. No treatment seemed to help, but when a magnetic applicator with less than one gauss of energy was placed on his solar plexus (a bundle of nerves located behind the stomach) for only three minutes, his symptoms immediately ceased. Two years later, Stan had experienced no relapse.

In another case, Ted, 70, had undergone coronary bypass surgery but continued to suffer from heart pain. His walk was reduced to a shuffle, his speech was slurred, and he lived in a state of chronic depression. Ted decided to try magnetic therapy in which a magnet was placed over his heart. Within ten minutes, the pain disappeared. Magnets were applied to the crown of his head while he slept and, within a month, his depression was gone, his speech was clear, and his walking returned to normal.

In other cases, magnets have helped to eliminate toothaches, periodontal disease, as well eradicate fungal infections like candidiasis. They have also helped to dissolve calcium deposits and kidney stones. Even symptoms of atherosclerosis have disappeared after 6-8 weeks of nightly exposure to a negative static magnetic field. Magnetic therapy has been shown to be particularly effective in reducing all forms of swelling, or edema.

There are numerous forms of magnetic field therapy, including static magnetic fields produced by natural or artificial magnets, and pulsating magnetic fields generated by electrical devices. The magnetic fields produced by magnets or electromagnetic generating devices are able to penetrate the human body and can affect the functioning of the nervous system, organs, and cells. Magnetic fields can stimulate metabolism and increase the amount of oxygen available to cells. When used properly, magnetic field therapy has no known harmful side effects.

Common Factors in Chronic Diseases

Acute maladaptive reactions and chronic degenerative diseases share a number of common factors, regardless of the specific condition. By addressing these underlying factors with magnet therapy, the conditions for chronic diseases, as well as the diseases themselves, will be eliminated.

Acid pH—Injuries as well as acute maladaptive reactions evoke high acidity and simultaneously register electromagnetic positive. When the pH in the body stays on the acid side for an extended period of time, a condition of acidosis occurs. Acidosis is a central factor in the degenerative disease process. Chronic degenerative diseases, such as cancer and Type II diabetes, are acute acidic reactions extended into chronic states.

My clinical experience has involved testing the pH of a sizable number of patients and their maladaptive reactions to environmental substances. This clinical work provided convincing evidence that pH consistently turns acidic during these reactions. This occurs within an hour or so of an acute reaction and is also present in chronic degenerative diseases. The acidity is local where the symptoms develop; this usually is but may not necessarily be reflected by an assessment of the blood pH. If present, the systemic evidence (blood pH) after a maladaptive reaction classically becomes corrected in two to three hours.

Hypoxia—There is always an oxygen-deficit state (hypoxia) when acidity is present, because molecular oxygen cannot remain free in an acid medium. Since molecular oxygen is necessary for human energy production, the development of hypoxia is central to the acute and chronic disease process.

Free Radicals—Based on years of clinical reports from around the world, it is evident that free radicals play a major role in the development of infectious and degenerative diseases, as well as in acute inflammatory reactions. Some commonly known sources of free-radical production are excessive sun exposure, tobacco smoke, and industrial pollution, as well as most maladaptive food, chemical, and inhalant reactions.

Reduced Ionized Calcium–Degenerative diseases also commonly show a reduced ionized calcium, which is usually related to maladaptive, acidic reactions. Calcium plays a major role in metabolic function, but in an acid medium, calcium becomes insoluble.

This reduced calcium is not necessarily related to a lack of calcium in the diet. It is more likely a result of maladaptive reactions to foods, chemicals, and inhalants, in which the pH becomes acidic.

Impaired Cellular Function—Acid-hypoxic conditions produce swollen cells (edema), which do not function properly. When cells become swollen, then DNA cellular repair does not occur, mutations develop, and cells lose their ability for normal metabolism, which leads to the development of degenerative diseases.

How Magnets Work Therapeutically

The negative magnetic field heals by alleviating these common disease factors. It alkalinizes tissues and releases oxygen from its bound state back to its molecular state. By returning tissues to a normal, healthy state, a negative magnetic field governs energy recovery, relieves inflammation, swelling, and other symptoms, and accelerates healing.

Robert O. Becker, M.D., demonstrated that the body concentrates a negative electromagnetic energy at the site of an injury for healing.[1] Dr. Becker detected that positive electromagnetic energy initially exists at the site of injury, followed by this negative electromagnetic signal for healing. If the body succeeds in sending enough negative magnetic energy to the site of an injury, such as a cancerous growth, then it will heal this lesion. However, in many cases, the body simply does not supply and maintain enough negative magnetic energy at the injury to facilitate healing. This is because the human body has some limitations—based on its own energy capacity—on how much negative magnetic energy it can generate.

Adding a negative magnetic field from a source outside the body can provide anti-stressful energy of sufficient strength for healing to occur, supplementing the body's effort to heal. The body is then not required to be the sole provider of negative magnetic energy to its injured area.

Dr. Becker documented that melatonin and growth hormone secretion in human subjects may be changed by exposure to an anti-stress static magnetic field.[2] Melatonin is the primary neurohormone in control of energy,[3] regulating tissue regeneration and the activation of hormones, enzymes, and antioxidants. Melatonin also has anti-aging, anti-infectious, and anti-tumor functions. Growth hormone is also an anabolic hormone, made only during sleep, that governs the healing and growth processes, the conversion of amino acids into proteins, and the metabolism of fat.[4] Dr. Becker observed that when a negative static magnetic field from an external magnet is placed over an injured area, the cells are supplied with the energy that enables healing to proceed.[5]

My clinical observations have established a number of other effects for magnetic therapy:

■ A negative magnetic field is required for healing in general, including cuts, bruises, broken bones, allergic reactions, infections, and inflammation.

■ A negative magnetic field normalizes pH, which prevents or relieves the symptoms of immunologic and non-immunologic sensitivities and addictive withdrawal symptoms.

■ The oxygenation of cells and tissues occurs in the presence of a negative magnetic field.

The Physiological Effects of Negative and Positive Magnetic Fields

Negative Magnetic Fields	Positive Magnetic Fields
pH normalizing	Acid producing
Oxygenating	Oxygen deficit producing
Resolves cellular edema	Evokes cellular edema
Usually reduces symptoms	Often exacerbates existing symptoms
Inhibits microorganism replication; slows down infections	Accelerates microorganism replication; speeds up infections
Biologically normalizing	Biologically disorganizing
Reduces pain and inflammation	Increases pain and inflammation
Governs rest, relaxation, and sleep	Governs wakefulness and action
Evokes anabolic hormone production—melatonin and growth hormone	Evokes catabolic hormone production
Clears metabolically produced toxins out of the body	Produces toxic by-products of metabolism
Eliminates free radicals	Produces free radicals
Slows down electrical activity of the brain	Speeds up electrical activity of the brain

Promotes Alkaline-Hyperoxia

A positive magnetic field produces acidity, which causes an oxygen deficit. Under these conditions of acid-hypoxia, infectious and degenerative diseases of all kinds flourish, the body becomes sick and develops many different symptoms. Moreover, as the acidity of the body rises, it becomes more difficult for cells to use oxygen normally.

On the other hand, a negative magnetic field supplies the necessary alkalinity, which supports the presence of molecular oxygen. A negative magnetic field also has a direct effect on the vascular system of the body, allowing more oxygen to be delivered to the tissues.

Accordingly, acid-hypoxia (high acidity and low oxygen) is a central condition in both degenerative diseases and acute symptoms from maladaptive reactions. In contrast, alkaline-hyperoxia (low acidity and high oxygen) is the biologically normal state needed for energy production, oxidoreductase enzyme function, defense against infection, detoxification, and overall healing. Exposing the body to a negative magnetic field produces a biological response of alkaline-hyperoxia, helping to reverse undesirable symptoms and degenerative diseases.

In essence, therefore, the negative magnetic field begins the healing process by changing the conditions of acid-hypoxia to alkaline-hyperoxia. As such, it alkalinizes tissues and releases oxygen from its bound state back to its molecular state. And by returning tissues to an oxygen-rich and health-promoting alkaline state, a negative magnetic field inhibits infectious microorganisms, detoxifies free radicals, facilitates cellular and DNA repair, relieves inflammation, swelling, and other symptoms, governs energy recovery, and thus accelerates healing in general.

Normalizes pH

Acid-hypoxia (high acidity and low oxygen) is a central condition in both degenerative diseases and acute symptoms from maladaptive reactions. In contrast, alkaline-hyperoxia (low acidity and high oxygen) is the biologically normal state needed for energy production, oxidoreductase enzyme function, defense against infection, detoxification, and overall healing. Exposing the body to a negative magnetic field produces a biological response of alkaline-hyperoxia, helping to reverse symptoms and degenerative diseases.

Short-term symptom reversal involves the following:

1) Normalizing the pH with bicarbonates such as sodium and potassium. Breathing oxygen sometimes adds another relieving agent, since oxygen becomes deficient in the acid state.

2) Taking antioxidants (SEE QUICK DEFINITION) such as vitamins A, C, and E, and beta carotene. When taken beyond their specific nutritional needs, these antioxidants serve as absorbents for free radicals, nullifying the inflammatory response

3) Exposing the symptom area to a negative magnetic field.

Activates Normal Cellular Energy Production

Adenosine triphosphate (ATP—SEE QUICK DEFINITION), the main fuel for cellular energy, is pro-

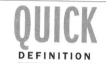

QUICK

DEFINITION

An **antioxidant** (meaning "against oxidation") is a natural biochemical substance that protects living cells against damage from harmful free radicals. Antioxidants work against the process of oxidation—the robbing of electrons from substances. If unblocked or left uncontrolled, oxidation can lead to cellular aging, degeneration, arthritis, heart disease, cancer, and other illnesses. Antioxidants in the body react readily with oxygen breakdown products and free radicals, and neutralize them before they can damage the body. Antioxidant nutrients include vitamins A, C, and E, beta carotene, selenium, coenzyme Q10, pycnogenol (grape seed extract), L-glutathione, superoxide dismutase, and bioflavonoids.

duced through a process called oxidation phosphorylation. During this process, molecular oxygen accepts an electron and becomes free radical oxygen (superoxide). If not immediately reversed enzymatically, superoxide proceeds to produce inflammatory free radicals, peroxides, oxyacids, alcohols, and aldehydes. The oxidoreductase family of enzymes has the assignment of making ATP as well as eliminating by-products of the oxidation process. These enzymes are dependent on alkalinity, oxygen, and activation by a negative magnetic field. If these three factors are not present, then cellular ATP is made by fermentation. This fermentation process is dependent on acidity and lack of oxygen—a positive magnetic field is necessary for this type of energy production, used by cancer cells and in other disease states.

A negative magnetic field facilitates the normal cellular production of ATP.[6] It is imperative to maintain an adequate negative static magnetic field, a normal alkaline body pH, and high levels of oxygen for maintaining health. Normal enzyme function is also dependent on the presence of certain nutrients in the body—see "Supplementing with Enzyme Cofactors," p. 33.

Releases Oxygen

A negative magnetic field supports the body's oxygenation in several ways. This is important because oxygen is necessary for ATP energy and oxidative remanent magnetism. Oxygen is also one of the body's defenses against disease, particularly against the development of local and systemic acidity. Oxygenation neutralizes acids that produce oxygen deficit, which predisposes the body to the development of degenerative disease. In addition, when supplied with abundant molecular oxygen, a favorable alkaline pH is maintained in the body. When acids exceed capacity, then oxygen is reduced and peroxides are formed, setting the groundwork for illness.

Many toxins that poison human enzyme systems are acids that have been oxidized. Oxygenation is the major detoxifying process for these toxins that threaten human health, including infectious microorganisms, peroxides, and free radicals. This requires an abundance of molecular oxygen (O_2) and an alkaline environment. A negative magnetic field supplies the necessary alkalinity, which supports the presence of oxygen.

Supplementing with Enzyme Cofactors

Enzyme function requires enzyme cofactors. The body synthesizes enzyme cofactors from essential nutrient precursors, but in the case of degenerative disease or with aging, this synthesis slows down or even stops. So, it may be wise to also supplement with enzyme cofactors, either as an initial functional boost of short duration or to be continued along with the negative magnetic field exposure. Consider the following coenzymes for supplementation:

■ NADH (nicotinamide adenine dinucleotide): The body makes NAD from niacinamide (vitamin B3). NAD is an essential enzyme cofactor in the oxidoreductase enzyme system. Nicotinamide is an essential electron transfer in the energy system and the production of adenosine triphosphate (ATP). As aging and other stress factors occur, the production of NAD diminishes, resulting in a loss of energy. Fortunately, NAD in its reduced form, NADH, is available as a nonprescription food supplement. Since NAD plays an important coenzyme function in the production of neurotransmitters, it is useful to supplement with NADH in neurotransmitter deficiency disorders, including chronic fatigue, depression, Parkinson's, Alzheimer's, and other degenerative diseases.[8] Typical recommended dose is 2.5 mg, three times per week or up to three times per day, depending on need (determined by the amount of NAD produced from vitamin B3).

■ Lipoic Acid: Lipoic acid serves the following functions: 1) acts as an antioxidant; 2) plays an essential role in energy production; 3) acts as a chelator, removing excess iron, copper, and toxic metals, such as cadmium, lead, and mercury; 4) normalizes blood sugar, helping to deter or reverse diabetes; 5) reduces protein damage, the rate of aging, and nerve damage, which occurs in diabetic neuropathy; 6) protects against DNA damage, heart disease, cancer, cataracts, and cellular deterioration; 7) improves neurological function and protects against nerve degeneration, which occurs in Parkinson's and Alzheimer's disease; and 8) decreases fat production.

Enzyme energy activation supports the production of lipoic acid, but when this production is sluggish, lipoic acid can be supplemented. In the case of serious degenerative disease and with aging, it may be wise to supplement for the first year of treatment. This can then be discontinued if negative magnetic field exposure during sleep maintains improved levels.[9] As a supplement, typically take 30 mg once or twice each day and one tablespoon of brewer's yeast, one or two times per day, each fourth day. Food sources include red meats and fish.

■ Coenzyme Q10: Coenzyme Q10 is a cofactor for the production of ATP. The body synthesizes coenzyme Q10 from nutritional vitamin precursors and a negative magnetic field energizes the body's synthesis of CoQ10. Coenzyme Q10 deficiency is a contributing factor in diabetes, obesity, reduced immune system function, reduced antioxidant function, aging, and heart disease. Typical recommended dose is up to 10 mg three times per day.

QUICK

Magnet therapy also has a direct effect on the vascular system of the body, allowing more oxygen to be delivered to the tissues.[7]

In contrast, detoxification cannot take place in an acid medium with insufficient oxygen. A positive magnetic field produces acidity, which causes an oxygen deficit. Under these conditions of acid-hypoxia, the body becomes sick and develops many symptoms. Also, as the acidity of the body rises, it becomes even more difficult for cells to use oxygen normally. Rather, molecular oxygen gets reduced into a bound state, and the oxidation process diminishes.

Eliminates Free Radicals

A negative magnetic field activates the oxidoreductase enzymes that reverse acids, hydrogen peroxide, and oxygen free radicals. As stated previously, this releases molecular oxygen, which is needed for oxidation.

Since a measurable magnetic field is present during oxidoreductase enzyme reactions, it is theoretically assumed that this field is the activation source. This theory is also based on the evidence that a positive magnetic field blocks the function of these enzymes. Without sufficient negative magnetic energy, these enzymes do not work to reverse the conditions that cause disease.

The oxidoreductase enzyme system also has the capacity to release oxygen and return it to its oxidatively useful molecular state. In addition, oxidoreductase enzymes process or reverse oxyacids and aldehydes, releasing molecular oxygen from its bound state in these often toxic substances. These by-products are formed when free radicals oxidize food substances and other organic compounds, such as petrochemicals.

When the load of free radicals exceeds the body's processing capacity, then the oxi-

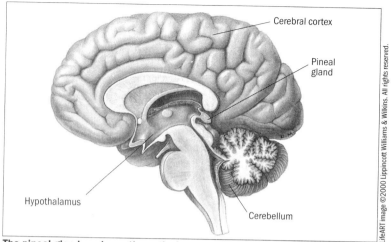

Cerebral cortex

Pineal gland

Hypothalamus

Cerebellum

The pineal gland produces the antioxidant hormone melatonin.

doreductase enzymes become inhibited. An external source of a negative magnetic field can energize these enzymes to quickly reduce free-radical production.[10]

Stimulates Hormone Production

Melatonin (SEE QUICK DEFINITION) secretion may be changed by exposure to a static magnetic field.[11] Melatonin has anti-aging, anti-infectious, and anti-cancer effects. Exposing the intestinal wall, pineal gland, and retina of the eyes to a static negative magnetic field stimulates the production of melatonin. Melatonin also reverses free radicals, including the hydroxyl radical.

Applying a static negative magnetic field over an area of cellular inflammation or degeneration produces the following: 1) a reversal of all free radicals; and 2) an activation of the bicarbonate buffer system, which produces a normal alkaline pH. Growth hormone (HGH—SEE QUICK DEFINITION) is also an anabolic hormone, made only during sleep, that governs the healing and growth processes, the conversion of amino acids into proteins, and the ability to burn fat.[12] Magnet therapy, by promoting sound sleep, stimulates the production of HGH.

Corrects Cellular Edema

The health of human cells depends on a higher ratio of potassium to

sodium inside the cell and a higher ratio of sodium to potassium outside the cell. This differential inside and outside the cell provides a
gradient that electrifies the cell membrane and enables its nutrient
and hormonal transport functions into and out of the cell (called the
sodium-potassium pump). This gradient difference also removes
water from inside the cell and prevents edema or excess swelling.
The action of the sodium-potassium pump is attributable to the
enzyme adenosine triphosphatase (ATPase), which controls the ratio
of potassium and sodium inside the cell. ATPase brings potassium
into the cell and discharges sodium. A negative magnetic field activates the ATPase enzyme and also provides the alkaline medium
needed for ATPase to work effectively.[13]

Negative magnetic field exposure also reverses or prevents cellular edema. Under these edema-free conditions, the transport functions of the cell membrane are physiologically normal. Local edema
can be resolved quickly by placing the affected area in a negative
magnetic field. Sleeping on a negative magnetic bed pad helps the
general function of the sodium-potassium pump throughout the
body.

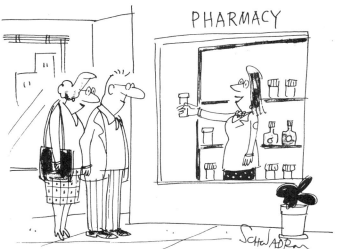

"THIS IS A REAL MIRACLE DRUG. IT COSTS THE SAME THIS YEAR AS IT DID LAST YEAR."

CHAPTER 3

Magnet Therapy in Practice

AGNETIC THERAPY can be applied in many ways, and devices range from small, simple magnets to large machines capable of generating high magnitudes of field strength. In regard to the magnets discussed in this book, specially designed ceramic, plastiform, and neodymium magnets can be placed either individually or in clusters above the organs of the body or on various points of the head. These types of magnets are commonly used because they are plate magnets with poles on opposite sides of flat surfaces, making it possible to expose the body to one magnetic field alone. Such a one-sided exposure, as previously stated, is the best way to use magnets, because most of the therapeutic value of magnetic therapy resides in the negative magnetic field.

For more about **magnet therapy for treating cancer**, see Cancer.

The strength of a magnet is measured in units of gauss—one gauss is equivalent to about twice the strength of the Earth's magnetic field. When considering the choice of therapeutic magnets, one must always consider a magnet's gauss strength in relation to its depth of penetration. For example, for a skin melanoma of less than 1" diameter, a 1" x $1/8$" neodymium magnet would be the magnet of choice, because the neodymium magnet's diameter is larger than the lesion being treated and the depth of its penetration is limited to approximately $1^1/_2$". On the other hand, for treating liver cancer, the right magnet would be either a 4" x 6" x $1/2$" or 4" x 6" x 1" ceramic magnet. This type of magnet has a negative magnetic field that pene-

A Quick Review of Magnet Basics

All magnets have two poles: positive (or "S" for south, usually marked in red) and negative (or "N" for north, usually marked in green). Negative magnetic energy normalizes and calms systems of the human body, while positive magnetic energy over-stimulates or disrupts the biological system. For this reason, negative poles are most frequently directed towards the body. Do not apply positive magnetic poles directly towards the body unless under medical supervision.

The most common types of magnets used in magnetic therapy are ceramic and neodymium (a rare earth chemical). These elements are mixed with iron to increase the magnet's strength or the duration of magnetic charge. The most powerful (and expensive) magnets are neodymium, while ceramic magnets are less expensive but still keep their charge for many years. These magnetic materials are incorporated into various types of products available at health food stores or through mail-order catalogs. Ceramic and neodymium mag-

nets are available as plastiform strips that attach to the skin by an elastic adhesive, wrist and back supports, seat pads, and strips worn inside shoes; magnetic blankets and beds are also available for promoting sleep and reducing stress.

The strength of a magnet is measured in gauss units (which measures the intensity of magnetic flux). Every magnetic device has a manufacturer's gauss rating; however, the actual strength of the magnet at the skin surface is often much less than this number. For example, a 4,000-gauss magnet transmits about 1,200 gauss to the patient. Magnets placed in pillow or bed pads will render even lower amounts of field strength at the skin surface, because a magnet's strength quickly decreases with the distance from the subject. The strength of the magnet also depends on its size and thickness. Therapeutic magnets use from 200 gauss to 1,500 gauss (only a fraction of what an MRI machine emits), while a common refrigerator magnet emits 10 gauss.[1]

trates from 4" to 6" and would be more appropriate than a neodymium magnet.

How to Use Magnets Therapeutically

Manufacturers of magnets rate the gauss strength of each magnet, but there is a difference when the magnet is used therapeutically. Specifically, when the magnet is placed directly on the body, you receive a lower level of gauss strength compared to the manufacturer's gauss rating. The further away the magnet, the weaker the magnetic field.

Ideally, a 25-gauss strength magnet or stronger should be used for the best therapeutic results. Always use the strongest magnet possible for achieving optimum treatment results. However, when selecting a specific magnet, consider not only the gauss rating of the magnet, but also the depth of its penetration in relation to the specific organ or part of the body being treated.

For example, a 4" x 4" x $\frac{1}{8}$" plastiform magnet provides about 50 gauss when applied directly on the surface of the body. Flexible magnet pads are made from small pieces of plastiform material. They are extremely flexible and light in weight, and provide a convenient form of magnetic treatment for many areas of the body. The 4" x 6" x $\frac{1}{2}$" ceramic magnet, on the other hand, provides approximately 280 gauss when applied directly on the surface of the body and has a greater depth of penetration than a plastiform magnet. Because of its depth of penetration, this particular type of magnet is a better choice for treating internal organs. The super neodymium magnet provides an extremely high gauss strength level, but its penetration is much weaker compared to the ceramic magnet. This magnet is ideal for treating skin problems of all kinds.

So, there are many factors to consider when selecting what type of magnet to use for the best therapeutic results, including the size of the magnet, its weight and convenience for placement, the strength of its gauss rating, and the depth of its penetration. All these factors make a significant difference and will in the end determine the effectiveness of the magnetic therapy.

Magnets can be stacked on top of each other by placing opposite poles together. The second magnet increases the gauss strength of the total by one-third, but each magnet added thereafter adds increasingly less strength. The optimum increase in magnetic field strength is reached at a stack of eight $\frac{1}{2}$" ceramic magnets. Practically speaking, when considering whether to stack magnets, one must always think about the additional weight involved—at some point, the additional weight and inconvenience nullifies the value of the increased gauss rating.

Flat-surfaced, plate magnets have opposite magnetic poles on opposite sides. Each opposite pole extends halfway through the magnet and meets the other in the middle, communicating at this "equator." If applying the negative side to the body, the only way to receive any of the positive field is if the magnet were pressed down far enough to extend beyond the equator at the side of the magnet. Placing the magnets close together and/or using padding can effectively prevent this problem.

It is important not to use magnets with both poles side-by-side on the same side. The positive pole is acidifying and produces an inflammatory

Magnetic Depth of Penetration

The following is a table of gauss strengths for a number of therapeutic magnets. The higher the gauss strength, the more therapeutic the magnet.

Magnet	Surface	1"	2"	3"	6"
14" x 25" Multipurpose Pad	324	40	15	12	8
4" x 6" x 1"	525	355	210	125	35
4" x 6" x ½"	280	180	112	70	23
1" x ⅛" Neodymium	1,250	86	15	5	—
Double Flex Mat	200	40	23	15	5
4" x 4" x ⅛" Plastiform	50	30	13	8	—
Two 4" x 4" x ⅛" Plastiform	100	68	34	13	—

reaction. The positive magnetic field excites microorganism replication and cancer cell growth; can cause seizures in a seizure-prone person if placed on the head; and can cause an irregular heartbeat in a person predisposed to such a condition if placed over the heart. A gauss meter can be used to demonstrate that no positive magnetic field extends beyond the edge of the magnet.

There are two ways to relieve pain with magnet therapy:

■ A positive magnetic field causes stress, which raises the level of endorphins, the body's own painkillers, and relieves pain.

■ A negative magnetic field is anti-stressful, replacing acid-hypoxia, which causes pain, with alkaline-hyperoxia, which relieves pain.

However, the only way to treat disease is to relieve acid-hypoxia by alkalinizing and oxygenating the tissues. Only the negative magnetic field can achieve this goal.

Local vs. Systemic Treatment

When considering local versus systemic negative field magnetic therapy, one must first understand paramagnetism. This refers to whether a substance has the ability to retain a magnetic field on a temporary or per-

Safe Uses of a Positive Magnetic Field

Even though the negative magnetic field is predominately the field of choice when treating most conditions, in some instances the positive magnetic field may be used. For example, a positive magnetic field can provide a spurt of energy at the beginning of the day. In order to accomplish this, briefly expose each adrenal gland in the morning to a positive magnetic field for three to five minutes to excite the production of catabolic hormones. Subsequently, one may expose the adrenal glands to a negative magnetic field for 30 minutes in the evening to achieve a calming effect.

In addition, a positive magnetic field can be used to excite neurons to function. Such a treatment is useful in cases of spinal cord injury (as in multiple sclerosis). In these cases, cells have undergone an "extinction of disuse," but are

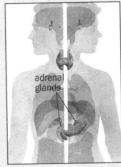

adrenal glands

still alive. Place a positive magnetic field over the symptomatic area and practice using the muscles or other functional parts to which the inhibited neurons relate. These 30-minute practice sessions involve brief positive magnetic field exposure in intervals of three minutes. After this brief exposure, continue practicing the muscle exercises in order to reinstate these neurons to their function. At the end of the session, place a negative magnetic field over the same area.

Those who have a latent potential for seizures, mental illness, or infections should completely avoid positive magnetic field exposures. This warning is especially true for exposures around the head, as this excites neurons and may make these conditions worse. Positive magnetic field exposure should only be used under medical supervision.

For more about **magnet therapy for treating multiple sclerosis**, see Multiple Sclerosis.

---

manent basis. The body has both paramagnetic and permanent magnetism. Permanent magnetism is present in the pineal gland, neurons, bones, and the ethmoid magnetic organ in the back of the nose. These organs contain magnetite crystals that retain a magnetic field permanently and bones are hard enough to retain magnetism on a permanent basis.

For more about **magnet therapy and infections**, see Infections.

Oxygen and water are also paramagnetic and it is possible to temporarily magnetize oxygen and water both externally and internally. Externally, these elements can be magnetized by exposure to a magnet, then taken into the body. Internally, when a permanent magnet is applied to an area of the body, the oxygen and water in that area become temporarily magnetized. This magnetized water and oxygen in the blood then flow from that local area to the entire body. When this occurs, the local treatment also has a systemic effect. This phenomenon accounts for many of the positive and indirect results of any negative field magnetic exposure.

Other forms of systemic treatment consist of sleeping on a magnetic bed pad along with placing a group of 4" x 6" x 1" magnets at the crown of the head. Such a nighttime exposure to the negative magnetic field oxygenates and alkalinizes the entire body. However, this systemic treatment should never be used in place of local treatment.

Local treatment consists of exposing a specific area of the body (joints, muscles, skin, internal organs) to a negative magnetic field. Magnets can also be applied to a cut, bruise, infection, or cancerous lesion. Minor disorders, such as bruises and cuts respond well to short-term negative magnetic field exposures. In the case of an infection or cancer, treatment must be continuous for much longer periods of time, with only minor breaks for bathing and one-hour breaks after meals to allow for digestion.

Specifically, infections should be treated 24-hours-a-day for a minimum of two weeks; cancer should be treated continuously for a minimum of 12 weeks. Remember that the negative magnetic field must be larger than the lesion being treated.

Types of Magnets

The magnets used in the therapy described in this book are permanent static field magnets with magnetic poles on opposite sides of flat surfaces. The negative magnetic pole side is usually marked with a green label ("N" or "-") and the positive magnetic pole side with a red label or "+".

Ceramic and
Neodymium Magnets

The ceramic iron oxide magnets and neodymium magnets are made of hard, non-flexible materials. These magnets hold their magnetic field permanently, with little loss over a period of many years. However, if dropped or allowed to snap together, this material will break or shatter. The following are examples of these magnets that are used in magnetic therapy:

■ $1^7/_8$" x $^7/_8$" x $^3/_8$" mini-block magnets: These are most often placed $1^1/_2$" apart in the bed pad, chair pad, or multipurpose pad. They can also be placed close together under a body wrap around joints or used to treat an infection either around a tooth or in the gums.

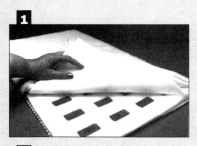

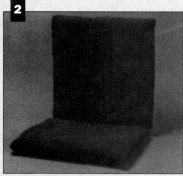

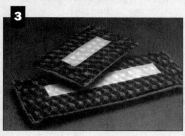

Magnets commonly used therapeutically include:
(1) Bed pad
(2) Comfort chair
(3) Flexible mats

■ $1^1/_2$" x $^1/_2$" ceramic magnet: Because of its strength and size, this magnet can be used to treat joints, muscles, tendons, and small infected areas or small cancerous lesions. For treatment of painful areas of joints, tendons, muscles, face, gums, and teeth, they can be used singly or close together. In order to increase the depth of penetration, these magnets can be placed on top of a multi-magnet flexible mat. For head treatment, the $1^1/_2$" x $^1/_2$" ceramic magnet should be placed bitemporally (on both temples) for most symptoms, including headaches, depression, or emotional upset.

■ 4" x 6" x $^1/_2$" ceramic block magnet: This magnet is one of the most widely used magnets. It is large enough to penetrate into the organs of the body and is often used on top of a flexible mat when treating the abdomen, lungs, liver, or spleen. This magnet is useful when placed against the side of the head during sleep, which increases the depth of sleep and also helps treat cerebral atherosclerosis.

■ 4" x 6" x 1" ceramic block magnets: These magnets are used in the Sleep Enhancer, where four of these magnets are placed in a row $^3/_4$" apart. In the super magnet bed, there are 70 of these magnets, placed 1" apart; this bed is useful for treating cancer and systemic infections. Since these magnets weigh four pounds each, they are seldom used around the body otherwise.

■ 2" x 5" x $^1/_2$" ceramic block magnet: Because of its size, it is very useful on smaller areas, particularly the wrist.

■ $^3/_4$" x $^1/_8$" ceramic disc magnet: It can be used on small areas, such as finger or toe joints, or lesions that are small enough to be covered. A number of magnetic bed pads are made from these magnets.

■ 1⅞" x ⅞" x ³⁄₈" mini-block magnet: It is ideal for treating finger or toe joints and several can be placed close together in a wrap around a joint, using as many as necessary. Since they can be taped to the face, directly over an infected tooth or gum, these magnets are especially useful in dentistry. The Mega-Field sleep pad contains these magnets.

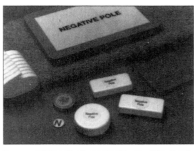

An assortment of magnets used in magnet therapy.

■ 1" x ⅛" neodymium disc magnet: This magnet is a hard ceramic material. Because it is small and lightweight, it can be taped to the body, strapped on with a band, or held in place by other magnets attached to the clothing. This magnet can be applied to the face over an infected tooth or gum, as long as the infected area is smaller than the magnet. It can also be used for treating small cancerous lesions or infections. Stacking these magnets increases gauss penetration.

For more about **magnet therapy for the skin**, see Skin Problems. For more about **magnet therapy for treating the eyes**, see Eye Problems.

■ ½" x ¹⁄₁₆" neodymium disc magnet: This type of magnet does not have as strong a gauss rating as a 1" x ⅛" magnet. This small magnet is useful for treating tiny lesions (less than ½" across), such as warts, moles, or small scars.

Flexible Plastiform Magnets

Plastiform magnets come in rolls that are 2", 3", or 4" wide and ⅛" thick and can be cut into any desired size. Common sizes are 2" x 2", 3" x 3", 4" x 4", 4" x 6", 4" x 12", 4" x 18", and 4" x 24". Cutting off the corners makes for greater comfort. Although they are flexible, these magnets will break if flexed a number of times. These magnets are approximately half as strong as the ceramic magnets that are ½" to 1" thick, but they are convenient to use for many purposes.

Their strength can be increased by stacking them. Four of these magnets stacked together have the equivalent gauss strength of a ½" ceramic magnet. If one plastiform magnet does not relieve the pain or inflammation, then stack two or three together to increase the gauss strength and depth of penetration into the tissues.

■ 4" x 6" x ⅛" plastiform strip: This plastiform magnet can be placed over muscle pains or skin lesions, on the lower back, or even over the heart.

■ 4" x 12" x ⅛" plastiform magnet: This magnet is commonly used for treating the spine and is especially useful when treating multiple sclerosis. Magnets on the spine can be 4" x 12", 4" x 18", or 4" x 24", depending on the need.

■ Double Magnet, Multi-Magnet Flexible Mat: This magnetic mat is composed of short strips of plastiform magnets that are held close together. The mat allows for increased flexibility, protects against breaking the magnets, and is useful for treatment around joints and curvatures of the body (especially the chest, abdomen, and shoulders). These mats come in 5" x 6" (equivalent to a 4" x 6" plastiform magnet) and 5" x 12" (equivalent to a 4" x 12" plastiform magnet) sizes and are encased in a nylon cover, which can be fastened to the clothing.

Other Magnets

■ Magnetic Eye Unit: This is composed of a magnetic light shield with 1" x ⅛" neodymium disc magnets placed directly over the eyes on the outside of the shield. For sinus treatment, the disc magnets can be placed over the sinuses.

■ Magnetic Head Unit: This is a wooden carrier (20" long) containing four 4" x 6" x 1" magnets stacked together on one side and a 4" x 6" x ½" magnet on the other side of the head (about 12" away).

■ Magnetic Cap: Neodymium discs in a cap that covers the entire head.

■ 70-Magnet Bed: Seventy 4" x 6" x 1" magnets placed 1" apart. Thirty-five magnets are placed in a sealed wooden carrier that measures 36" x 36"; two of these placed together forms the single-sized bed.

■ Mega-Field Magnetic Sleep Pad: This magnetic sleep pad is composed of 1⅞" x ⅞" x ⅜" mini-block magnets placed 1½" apart throughout the pad. It can be used on top of the mattress.

■ The Vitality Sleep Enhancer: This group of magnets is composed of four 4" x 6" x 1" magnets placed ¾" apart in a wooden carrier. A shelf between the mattress and springs holds this carrier firmly against the headboard so it cannot tip. These magnets can be raised or lowered, depending on the height of the pillow. Place the carrier so the bottom of the magnets are level with the back of the head.

How to Apply Magnets

The use of various fabric wraps is the most popular and efficient method of fastening magnets on the body. One of the most useful is a fabric wrap, which comes in two sizes: 2" x 26" and 4" x 52". The 2" x 26" wrap is adjustable and is commonly used around the head. A strip of Velcro on the positive field side of a magnet can be used to attach the magnet to the fabric. A 4" x 52" fabric wrap can be used on the abdomen and pelvic area.

When using large and heavy magnets, make a garment of non-stretchable material that will drape from the shoulders, designed with appropriate magnet-sized pockets fitting directly over the areas to be treated.

Tubular elastic dressing retainers from a medical supply store come in all sizes and are suitable for holding magnets on a finger, arm, leg, or the trunk of the body. A magnet can be held under the elastic bandage with self-adhesive wrap. Braces for various areas of the body are also available at medical supply stores. These braces can be used to treat the neck, back, wrist, or shoulders, with the magnet attached either under or on the outside of these supports. Magnets can be placed on the outside of either a soft or hard cast; the magnetic field will go directly through the cast. Suitable magnets to place over a cast include the $\frac{1}{2}$" ceramic magnets, which can be sized for the area being treated.

Some people prefer to attach small magnets directly on the skin. This can be achieved by using a skin tape (such as Elastikon by Johnson & Johnson and Coban by 3M) readily available at any drugstore. Either of these can satisfactorily hold a small magnet in place on the skin. For those people who are sensitive to skin tape, there are other hypoallergenic tapes available (such as HY tape). Another useful way of holding magnets in place is to attach them to the body with elastic ACE bandages. The magnets can be placed within an ACE bandage and then wrapped in place. In addition, a spot-type Band-Aid can be used to hold the $\frac{1}{2}$" neodymium magnet directly on the skin over a small lesion.

Precautions When Using Magnets

The following guidelines should be implemented whenever magnetic therapy is considered as a treatment modality:

■ Do not use magnets over the uterus during pregnancy. There is no known harm, but also no published data.

■ The usual response to a negative magnetic field bed pad is an increased ability to relax, deeper sleep, and vivid dreams. Occasionally, a

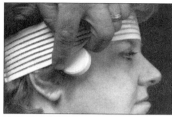

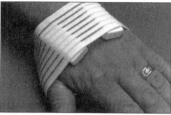

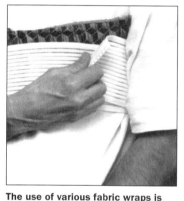

The use of various fabric wraps is the most popular and efficient method of fastening magnets on the body:
(Top) Temporal wrap
(Middle) Miniblocks wrapped around the wrist
(Bottom) Chest wrap

person will complain of lethargy, usually the result of improving their ability to relax. Maintain exposure up to tolerance and, in a few days, these symptoms should be relieved through normal detoxification.

■ In order not to interfere with proper digestion, always wait 60-90 minutes after meals before applying magnetic therapy to the upper abdomen.

■ Do not apply the positive magnetic field unless under direct medical supervision. It can produce seizures, hallucinations, insomnia, and hyperactivity, stimulate the growth of tumors and microorganisms, as well as promote addictive behavior.

■ A negative magnetic field pulls interstitial fluid (located between the cells) toward the field. At the same time, it pulls fluid out of the cells and into the interstitial space. This fluid increase in a closed, non-draining area may cause pain. Eventually, the pain will be reduced or eliminated because a negative magnetic field will cancel out the underlying cause of the excessive fluid, namely infection or inflammation.

■ Occasionally, paresthesias develop around the area of a lesion that is being treated with a negative magnetic field. Paresthesias are odd, low-intensity sensations that differ from person to person, described variously as burning, itching, aching, tingling, feeling hot or cold, or even occasional pain. These symptoms are most likely to occur when there is a prolonged magnetic exposure and are usually fleeting. Stroking the skin or vibration may stop the paresthesia and there will be no need to remove the magnet.

Part Two

An A-Z of Health Conditions with Magnet Therapy Success Stories

Addictions

ADDICTION CAN BE DEFINED as any physical or psychological dependence that negatively impacts a person's life. Although a person can be addicted to many forms of behavior, such as gambling, over-eating, sex, or reckless behavior, the term *addiction* is most commonly used to refer to dependency on cigarettes, alcohol, and drugs (both legal and illegal). In severe cases, addiction can become so obsessive that it may seem to take on a life of its own, and the individual's true identity can take a second place to the personality of the addiction.

It is also possible to become addicted to any food eaten as frequently as twice a week. Narcotic addiction refers to being addicted to such substances as cocaine, morphine, or heroin. When exposed to a narcotic, the person feels physically and mentally euphoric, pain-free, and concern-free. Three to four hours after exposure, a withdrawal phase sets in. The body manufactures its own narcotics, neurotransmitters called endorphins, in response to the stress of a frequently eaten food or chemical contact, such as from tobacco or caffeine. These self-made narcotics can be just as addictive. Withdrawal occurs when there is a significant drop in either the external or internal narcotic. In withdrawal, the person becomes depressed, weak, agitated, or experiences pain.

All narcotics, whether produced in the body or taken externally, are alkaloids. As such, they initially raise the body's pH to an alkaline state to make oxygen available. However, when the withdrawal phase sets in, a combination of high acidity and low levels of oxygen occurs. Addictions are thus characterized by a seesaw effect between these states of alkaline-hyperoxia and acid-hypoxia. Withdrawal symptoms develop as a result of too much acidity and low oxygen levels (acid-hypoxia) in the body. The negative magnetic field can reverse this undesirable metabolic state and change it into a more health-promoting state that supplies alkalinity and oxygen to all cells.

The addictive process also produces positive magnetic field stimulation of the brain and body. Stress is relieved by the body by the release of the neurotransmitter serotonin (SEE QUICK DEFINITION) and endorphins, which are natural opiates produced by the body. But in a state of chronic stress, the body is no longer able to produce enough serotonin or endorphins. This sets the stage for food addictions. Foods are eaten that trigger the release of the serotonin, but at levels higher than normal, often leading to higher blood sugar levels and impaired mental functioning. Foods are thus being used as a drug to relieve symptoms and, like a drug, you can become addicted to them.

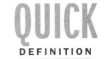

QUICK
DEFINITION

Serotonin is a neurotransmitter, a brain chemical with the specific function of enabling communications between brain cells, called neurons. Electrical thought impulses are changed into neurotransmitters at the dendrites, the branching tips of a nerve cell; then they are passed on to the next nerve cell. Serotonin is a calming agent that works to stop excess nerve signals (stimulation) and thus keeps brain firings from getting out of control. It helps produce sleep, regulate pain, and influence mood—it's called the "feel good" neurotransmitter—although too much serotonin can produce depression.

This metabolic roller coaster of addiction leads to an eventual burnout of metabolic functions and a collapse of health. Fortunately, this overdrive can be reduced with sufficient negative magnetic field exposure, which normalizes the functions of the body and brain. In particular, a negative magnetic field helps to stop the addictive craving for a particular narcotic substance and helps to relieve withdrawal symptoms.

Treatment Options for Addictions

It is important to stop all addictions at the same time, whether it is to narcotics, tobacco, alcohol, caffeine, or foods. To prevent and treat food addictions, avoid any food eaten as frequently as two or more times a week. This includes the entire food family to which the specific food belongs. For example, if addicted to gluten, any cereal grain containing gluten (wheat, rye, oats, and barley) needs to be withheld from the diet. In addition, a number of commonly used alcoholic beverages are made from these gluten-bearing cereal grains.

For the **Four-Day Diversified Rotation Diet**, see Appendix.

Gluten-containing cereal grains lead to the highest number of maladaptive reactions to foods. These frequently used foods, including their family members, should be avoided for at least three months. They can then be reintroduced into the diet using a Four-Day Diversified Rotation Diet.

Magnet Therapy

When treating addictions, one must totally avoid the use of all addictive substances and should spend up to 30 minutes per day using magnets for symptom relief whenever withdrawal symptoms occur. Withdrawal symptoms will usually be relieved in this manner within 10-30 minutes.

Left temporal and low occipital (back of the head) placement of magnets is especially useful for addicts, as is left temporal and mid-forehead placement. Bitemporal placement (in front of and near the top of the ears) is another useful placement. Use either two $1^1/_2$" x $^1/_2$" ceramic disc magnets or two 1" x $^1/_8$" neodymium disc magnets. These magnets can be worn continuously over the temples, but should at minimum be used when withdrawal symptoms begin. In addition, place a 4" x 6" x $^1/_2$" ceramic magnet lengthwise on the sternum (mid-chest), and place a 4" x 6" x $^1/_2$" ceramic magnet over the epigastric area (upper abdomen, just below the sternum). These magnets should be left in place long enough to alleviate symptoms. The longer the exposure, the better.

Treating the spine with magnets provides an additional therapeutic value. Use either a 4" x 12" or a 4" x 24" plastiform magnet, or a 5" x 12" double magnet, flexible magnetic mat made from plastiform strips (these mats should be placed on the upper back in the thoracic area as well as on the lumbar area).

Placing magnets over the liver can facilitate detoxification. First, place a 5" x 12" double magnet, multi-magnet flexible mat across the front and side of the body over the liver. Next, place a 4" x 6" x $^1/_2$" magnet on either the side or front of the body, or on both areas, directly on top of the flexible mat. This added magnetic field will penetrate deeply into the liver, providing extra oxygen and normalizing pH. A 4" x 52" body wrap can be used to hold these magnets in place. Some people find it better to make a garment supported from the shoulders that has pockets to hold these magnets in place over the liver. It is best to wear this magnet garment over the liver 24 hours a day. The one exception to this rule is to withhold magnetic exposure for one hour after each meal in order for digestion to occur.

The addictive withdrawal phase is characterized by spasm of the muscles of the gastrointestinal tract (esophagus, stomach, and small and large intestines). Wherever this type of spasm occurs, place a negative magnetic field over the area to stop the spasm. It is also important to treat any painful areas with appropriate negative magnetic field exposure (remember that the size of the magnet must be larger than the area being treated).

It requires four to five days to work through the withdrawal phase of a food or alcohol addiction. However, since the alcoholic is often quite toxic, liver treatment needs to be extended anywhere from several days to one month. Tobacco addiction is somewhat different, in that nicotine is fat-soluble. It takes 20-30 days for fat cells to eliminate nicotine and some withdrawal symptoms will occur during this time period.

For more on **treating pain with magnets**, see Pain.

Nutritional Supplementation

While magnets can alleviate addictive withdrawal symptoms without additional support, the use of nutritional supplements can also be helpful. Vitamin C, vitamin B complex, and the minerals calcium and magnesium (in doses twice the recommended daily allowance) can provide relief for those interested in self-help options. In boosting the body's biochemical defenses against addiction, Janice Keller Phelps, M.D., uses nutritional supplements and adrenal supports, such as vitamin C, pantothenic acid (vitamin B5), and adrenal extracts in her treatment regimen. She also stresses that a patient must remove all addictive substances from the diet, including sugar and caffeine.

Megavitamin therapy is commonly cited as one of the most vital tools for replenishing vitamin deficiency, which affects more than 50% of all alcoholics. Narcotics addicts often suffer from a deficiency of essential minerals, especially magnesium, calcium, and potassium. Since alcohol enhances free-radical formation (the molecules held responsible for damaging and possibly aging the body), antioxidants are needed to oppose their effects, such as selenium, zinc, and vitamins C and E. Chromium aids in stabilizing the erratic blood sugar seen in alcoholic hypoglycemia, while choline and folic acid are also commonly cited as important supplements to assist in the body's recovery from addiction.

For more on **food addictions**, see *Weight Loss: An Alternative Medicine Definitive Guide* (Alternative Medicine.com Books, 2000; ISBN 1-887299-19-X); to order, call 800-333-HEAL.

Intravenous withdrawal support for severe cases is often used by James Braly, M.D. He states that those with severe withdrawal problems can benefit from three or four consecutive days of intravenous therapy consisting of vitamin C, calcium gluconate, magnesium sulfate, pantothenic acid, and vitamin B6. "Withdrawal symptoms can often be completely eliminated after one or two days using this approach," Dr. Braly says. Other nutrients that he recommends include evening primrose oil, vitamin B complex, and glutamine (an amino acid).

Alzheimer's Disease

ALZHEIMER'S DISEASE IS a progressive, degenerative disease that attacks the brain, resulting in impaired memory, decreased intellectual and emotional functioning, and ultimately complete physical breakdown. It was first identified in 1907 by German physician Alois Alzheimer who, during postmortem examinations, discovered abnormal formations of plaque on nerve endings and tangles of nerve fibers in the brain tissue of individuals who had exhibited symptoms of senile dementia. This plaque (amyloid) was found primarily in the hippocampus, the part of the brain related to memory and intellectual function.

Alzheimer's disease is the most common form of senile dementia, afflicting approximately 10% of those over the age of 65 and almost 50% of those over the age of 85.[1] Symptoms vary from depression, fatigue, and occasional forgetfulness to disorientation and aggressive or paranoid behavior. This range of symptoms, coupled with the fact that a definite diagnosis can be obtained only in postmortem examination, causes frequent misdiagnosis.

What Causes Alzheimer's?

Alzheimer's research is beginning to uncover multiple factors that may contribute to the disease. This indicates that the search for a single cause may be unfounded. Possible contributing factors include genetic tendencies, as well as environmental influences and nutritional deficiencies.

The common denominator of amyloidosis (the formation of amyloid plaque) is the disordered metabolism of the target area. These areas have the highest levels of acidity and the lowest levels of oxygen (acid-hypoxia). In such an environment, calcium in body fluids turns into crystals and amino acids become insoluble gels or deposits of amyloid.[2] In contrast, when a normal alkaline state, rich in oxygen, is maintained in the body, minerals and amino acids remain soluble.

Any factor that produces acid-hypoxia predisposes a person to the development of Alzheimer's disease. These factors include chronic degenerative diseases such as diabetes, infections, inflammation, atherosclerosis, addiction, and other toxic states. There is a central degenerative disease process in amyloidosis, diabetes, and atherosclerosis,[3] namely, chronic maladaptive food, chemical, and inhalant reactions that produce high acidity and low levels of oxygen in the body.

Genetic Tendencies—Researchers have discovered a link between genetic predisposition and Alzheimer's disease. In many families, people in succeeding generations develop Alzheimer's. A specific connection has also been uncovered between Alzheimer's and Down syndrome (a variety of mental retardation). Individuals suffering from Down syndrome often exhibit Alzheimer's-like memory problems or dementia in their thirties and forties. Postmortem examinations of the brains of older Down patients have revealed many of the characteristic abnormalities of Alzheimer's, such as nerve plaques and nerve fiber tangles in the brain.[4]

Environmental Influences—Gary Oberg, M.D., past President of the American Academy of Environmental Medicine, treats patients suffering from environmental illness. "Toxins such as chemicals in food and tap water, carbon monoxide, diesel fumes, solvents, aerosol sprays, and industrial chemicals can cause symptoms of brain dysfunction which may lead to an inaccurate diagnosis of Alzheimer's or senile dementia," says Dr. Oberg.

Studies have shown that a susceptibility to toxins such as aluminum and mercury are linked to the onset of Alzheimer's and senile dementia. Research indicates that, because of the high levels of aluminum found in the brain cells of Alzheimer's victims, this metal may be a causal factor in the development of the disease. While the source of aluminum toxicity in the body has not yet been proven, aluminum can enter the body through inhalation (by factory workers in certain industries) and by oral ingestion. It has been suggested that aluminum ions may leach into the body from aluminum cooking utensils, cans, and foil, as well as underarm deodorants, antacid pills, and other common products, many of which contain traces of aluminum.[5]

A study involving postmortem examination of brain tissue from Alzheimer's victims has also indicated the presence of high levels of mercury.[6] Another study makes a clear connection between the presence of mercury in brain tissue and the presence of "silver" amalgam dental fillings, which contain approximately 50% mercury as well as silver, tin, copper, and zinc.[7]

"In a recent test of 7,000 patients, we found 90.3% to be sensitive to mercury," says Hal A. Huggins, D.D.S., of Colorado Springs, Colorado. "What this means is, that while different people will react in different ways to mercury, in 90.3% of the people with amalgam fillings, the mercury will significantly suppress the immune system." Reactions to high levels of mercury in the body can range from nervousness and depression to suicidal tendencies and severe neurological diseases such as multiple sclerosis, Lou Gehrig's disease (a syndrome marked by muscular weakness and atrophy due to degeneration of motor neurons of the spinal cord, medulla, and cortex), and Alzheimer's. There is a relationship between Alzheimer's disease and high levels of ammonia in the body.[8] Ammonia is highly neurotoxic and can cause neuron death.

My clinical experience has brought me to the conclusion that mercury and aluminum toxicity is not the cause of Alzheimer's or Lou Gehrig's disease. These metals accumulate because dead neurons cannot process them out of the body.

Nutritional Deficiencies—Reduced levels of certain vitamins, minerals, and amino acids have been tentatively linked with Alzheimer's,[9] including folic acid, niacin (vitamin B3), thiamine (vitamin B1), vitamin B6, vitamin B12, vitamin C, vitamin D, vitamin E, magnesium, selenium, zinc, and tryptophan.

Treatment Options for Alzheimer's

The appropriate program for Alzheimer's disease is to first adequately handle all factors producing acid-hypoxia. Commonly used foods and chemicals should be avoided for five days. This prepares the way for allergy testing of foods and chemicals (see your practitioner). After the completion of this testing, a Four-Day Diversified Rotation Diet is recommended. Also, you must strictly avoid all chemicals to which you reacted.

For the **Four-Day Diversified Rotation Diet**, see Appendix.

Laboratory assessment of vitamin, mineral, amino acid, and essential fatty acid levels should also be done and any nutritional deficiencies should be treated accordingly. Optimum nutrition can help to eliminate the toxic metals that have accumulated in the brain and body of the person with Alzheimer's. Sources of heavy metal toxicity should also be avoided. The presence of lead, aluminum, and mercury deserves special laboratory assessment—if present, these toxic substances should be removed from the body by chelation (SEE QUICK DEFINITION).

You should consider removing silver-mercury amalgams from the teeth. I have seen numerous patients who simply could not reverse their mental or physical degenerative disease until their amalgams were removed. Using chelation immediately after amalgam removal can prevent undesirable side effects.

It is important to have a laboratory assessment of any possible infections, particularly viruses such as Epstein-Barr, cytomegalo, and human herpes virus #6. These viruses infect the neurons of the brain and spinal cord and they can be assessed by their antibody presence in the blood. Moreover, *Candida* infection and any possible bacterial infections should also be assessed.

QUICK DEFINITION

Chelation therapy refers to a method of binding up ("chelating") toxins (e.g., heavy metals) and metabolic wastes and removing them from the body while at the same time increasing blood flow and removing arterial plaque. One type of chelation therapy involves the chelating agent disodium EDTA given as an intravenous infusion over a 3½ hour period. Usually 20 to 30 treatments are administered at the rate of one to three sessions per week. Chelation therapy is especially beneficial for all forms of atherosclerotic cardiovascular disease including angina pectoris and coronary artery disease.

For more about **magnet therapy and infections**, see Infections.

Magnet Therapy

The acidity and lack of oxygen associated with Alzheimer's can be corrected with exposure to a negative magnetic field to produce an alkaline-hyperoxic response. A prolonged magnetic exposure will eventually reverse acid-hypoxia, and the amino acids and crystallized calcium will slowly return to their normal state. The amyloid plaque, composed of insoluble amino acids and calcium, becomes soluble in an alkaline medium.

On the other hand, a brief negative magnetic field exposure to the head does sometimes produce an observable reduction in some of the mental symptoms associated with Alzheimer's within ten to 30 minutes.[10] For example, Mary, a woman in her sixties, was disoriented due to her Alzheimer's disease. Within ten minutes of a negative magnetic field exposure to her head, she was mentally clear. The magnetic field was then removed and she retained her mental clarity for several hours. One clinical study found that a brief exposure to an extremely low frequency electromagnetic field improved visual memory as well as cognitive functions and energy levels in two Alzheimer's patients.[11]

A negative magnetic field can help in the detoxification process for those with Alzheimer's. By alkalinizing and activating the oxidoreductase enzymes, toxins involved in Alzheimer's, including the heavy metals mercury and aluminum, are processed for elimination from the body.

When considering magnetic therapy, expect the magnetic treatment to take several months in order to resolve the amyloid deposits. At the same time, use systemic treatment by sleeping on a negative magnetic bed pad and with magnets at the crown of the head.

For local treatment, use the magnetic head unit, consisting of a wooden carrier containing four 4" x 6" x 1" magnets stacked and one 4" x 6" x $^1/_2$" magnet. Sleep using this magnetic head unit at night and during daytime naps.

Place the negative field of a 5" x 12" double magnet, multi-magnet flexible mat with six mini-blocks directly over the heart and chest. This procedure magnetizes the oxygen and water flowing through the heart and dissolves any fat or amyloid plaques in the heart. This magnet over the heart can be held in place with the same body wrap that holds the magnets on the chest. The more hours of exposure to the negative magnetic field over the chest and heart, the better. It is preferable to maintain exposure 24 hours a day.

For depression and serious mental reactions, place the ceramic magnets bitemporally (in front of and at the top of the ears) held in place with a body wrap. For anxiety, first place one disc on the midforehead. Then, for a left-handed person, place the other over the right temporal area; for a right-handed person, place the other over the left temporal area.

For obsessive-compulsiveness, place the discs on the left temporal and occipital (base of the skull) areas. The longer the exposure to the magnetic field, the better will be the results.

In addition, sleep on a negative magnetic bed pad. This bed pad is composed of $1^7/_8$" x $^7/_8$" x $^3/_8$" mini-block magnets, placed $1^1/_2$" apart throughout the pad. The magnetic bed, composed of 70 4" x 6" x 1" magnets placed 1" apart, can also be used.

Oxygen and water can be magnetized in various ways and used for treatment of Alzheimer's. This can be achieved by using an oxygen concentrator and oxygen magnetizer. An oxygen concentrator supplies oxygen and the oxygen magnetizer exposes the oxygen to the negative magnetic field of a ceramic magnet. The result is magnetized oxygen. Breathe the oxygen during sleep and four times during the day for one hour each time.

Nutritional Supplements

Nutritional supplementation offers additional support in treating Alzheimer's. Studies in Japan have shown that daily supplements of coenzyme Q10, vitamin B6, and iron returned some Alzheimer's-diagnosed patients to "normal" mental capacity.[12] In another study, Alzheimer's patients who took a daily regimen of evening primrose oil, zinc, and selenium showed significant improvements in alertness, mood, and mental ability.[13]

Orthomolecular physician Abram Hoffer, M.D., combines niacin, which improves circulation and lowers cholesterol levels, with large doses of vitamins C and E. He also recommends folic acid, noting that 40% of all senile patients are deficient in this B vitamin.

Sandra Denton, M.D., of Anchorage, Alaska, also uses a program of nutritional supplements to build the immune systems of Alzheimer's patients and those with senile dementia. Her program is based on individual need and normally includes vitamins C, E, and B12 to increase circulation in the brain. Dr. Denton notes that many chronic health conditions improve once the gastrointestinal tract regains its functional integrity. She also stresses the importance of maintaining healthy function of the gastrointestinal tract in order to ensure proper vitamin and mineral absorption.

Chelation Therapy

Garry F. Gordon, M.D., co-founder of the American College of Advancement in Medicine, reports that chelation therapy can benefit memory in patients with Alzheimer's-like dementia by improving blood flow to the brain. However, magnet therapy is superior to chelation for resolving the insoluble amino acid and calcium deposits in Alzheimer's.

Chelation therapy uses chelating agents (such as EDTA—ethylenediaminetetraacetic acid) administered intravenously to restore proper circulation by removing the calcium content of plaque from arterial walls. Dr. Gordon cites numerous studies showing an increase in cerebrovascular circulation using EDTA chelation therapy.[14] Chelation therapy may also be beneficial to patients with senile dementia by removing aluminum, mercury, and other heavy metals from the body.

For more on **chelation**, see *Alternative Medicine Guide to Heart Disease* (Future Medicine Publishing, 1998; ISBN 1-887299-10-6); to order, call 800-333-HEAL.

For more about **magnet therapy and atherosclerosis**, see Heart Disease.

Charles Farr, M.D., Ph.D., co-founder of the American Board of Chelation Therapy, uses chelation therapy in cases of senile dementia that are due to either atherosclerosis (hardening of the arteries) of the cerebral arteries or toxins in the body. "When a patient comes in and is not functioning well, having trouble concentrating and remembering things, we have no immediate way of measuring whether it is a circulatory problem, toxicity, or an Alzheimer's-like situation." In cases of senile dementia, Dr. Farr recommends ten to 15 chelation treatments in order to more quickly stimulate the circulatory system. If the patient has atherosclerosis or is suffering from environmental toxins, a turnaround by 15 treatments is expected. If not, Dr. Farr assumes it is Alzheimer's.

Cancer

CANCER IS A DISEASE process in which healthy cells stop functioning and maturing properly. A mishap occurs inside these cells. Perhaps it begins with a change (mutation) in the genetic blueprint, its DNA. The altered DNA makes copies of itself and passes its information and gene sequencing on to other cells, which then become cancer prone. As the normal cycle of cell creation and death is interrupted, the newly mutated cancer cells begin multiplying uncontrollably, no longer operating as an integrated and harmonious part of the body.

In its simplest terms, cancer represents an accelerating process of inappropriate, uncontrolled cell growth—a chaotic process within the order of biology. Cancer cells, when examined under a microscope, are abnormally shaped, inconsistently formed, and disorganized and contain misshapen internal structures—the essence of biological disorder.

Cancer may seem to us a modern epidemic, but traces of cancer have been detected in the bones and skulls of mummies from Egypt and Peru embalmed 5,000 years ago. Hippocrates (circa 400 B.C.), the renowned Greek physician, first coined the term *carcinoma* to indicate skin cancer; to him, this Greek word (*karkinoma* means "crab") is appropriate because of the way a spreading cancer extends clawlike extensions across the cell, tissue, or skin. What is different today is the incidence of cancer: it is steadily affecting more people each year, specifically one out of every three. It is no longer one serious disease among many, but the disease of our time.

The development and growth of a cancer is called carcinogenesis. Physicians now understand that it involves many steps,

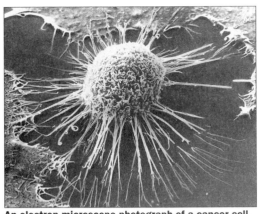
An electron microscope photograph of a cancer cell.

beginning with specific, undesirable changes in the nucleus of the cell, specifically in its genetic components, the DNA. What distinguishes a cancer process from life-as-usual in the cell is that normally—in a state of health—DNA mutations are repaired or rendered harmless by the immune system, an intricate, multifaceted biochemical defense system. When undesirable genetic alterations remain uncorrected, then a cancer process can potentially escalate to its next stage of uncontrolled rapid growth. It does this by making copies of itself. This replication, again, is a normal function of DNA, but the trouble here is that it is altered, mutated, and undesirable DNA that is copying itself. As more cancer cells are generated, the process continues to expand and form a tumor. The normal mechanisms of cell growth, replication, differentiation, and maturation then become unregulated, leading to chaos in the body.

The number of new cancers reported annually has increased steadily since the 1960s, as have cancer-related mortality rates for a variety of cancers. In 1900, a mere 3% of deaths were attributed to cancer, yet today, that number has jumped by eight times—to 24%. To put this in perspective, this is an 800% increase in less than a century. The National Cancer Institute reports a 28% rise in the incidence of childhood cancers from 1950 to 1988. Against some of the more common cancers in the United States—lung, liver pancreas, brain, and bone, as well as advanced cancers of the colon, breast, and prostate—little or no progress has been made in conventional medicine's expensive "War on Cancer," since it was declared in 1971 by then-president Richard Nixon.

Cancer is the number one health concern of every American, and for good reason. Each year, about 1.3 million people in the U.S. will be diagnosed with cancer and more than half this number will probably die from the disease or its treatment. That's about one American life lost to cancer every 45 seconds. "Despite some gains, cancer death rates remain unacceptably high, and the disease will kill 554,740 people in the U.S. this year," wrote J. Madeleine Nash in a special edition of *Time* magazine that summarized conventional cancer treatments.[1] Cancer now kills more children between the ages of 3 and 14 than any other illness.[2] Of greater concern is the fact that the numbers of both new cancer cases and deaths continue to rise. From 1950 to 1980, there was an 8% increase in cancer deaths,[3] but from 1975 to 1989, the number of new cancer cases reported each year increased 13% and the mortality rate rose 7%.[4] Although mortality rates for a few less-common cancers declined, overall rates have continued to rise.[5]

According to John C. Bailar III, Ph.D., professor of epidemiology and biostatistics at McGill University in Toronto, Canada, conventional medicine is decidedly losing the war on cancer. In 1993, he declared: "In the end, any claim of major success against cancer must be reconciled with this figure," referring to the steady increase in cancer deaths between 1950 and 1990. "I do not think such reconciliation is possible and again conclude [as he had in 1986 when making a similar retrospective review of data] that our decades of war against cancer have been a qualified failure. Whatever we have been doing, it has not dealt with the broadly rising trend in mortality."[6]

What Causes Cancer?

Conventional medicine's investigation into the causes of all forms of cancer has primarily focused on how specific carcinogens damage the DNA within healthy human cells. Medicine's preoccupation with this area of research has continued because the development of cancer always involves injury to the DNA of specific cells in the body. Due to our modern exposure to various carcinogenic chemicals and inhalants, we literally receive thousands of injuries to this DNA genetic material in the course of a day. And these carcinogens injure human DNA in such a dramatic way that breaks occur in this genetic material. Tumors arise as a result of a series of these breaks, changes, or rearrangements in the information coded within the DNA of damaged cells.

The alternative view of what causes cancer diverges from the widely held conventional research focus on a single precipitating cause. Rather, it points to multiple factors, both internal and external, which, in combination, over time contribute to a disease process in a given individual. These factors—ranging from environmental toxins and food additives to chronic stress and genetic predisposition—together

For more on the **causes of cancer**, see *Alternative Medicine Definitive Guide to Cancer* (Future Medicine Publishing, 1997; ISBN 1-887299-01-7); to order, call 800-333-HEAL.

Factors That Contribute to Cancer

- Sunlight
- Geopathic Stress
- Ionizing Radiation
- Industrial Toxins
- Polluted Water
- Fluoridated Water
- Hormone Therapies
- Irradiated Foods
- Mercury Toxicity
- Nerve Interference Fields
- Chronic Stress
- Depressed Thyroid Action
- Parasites
- Free Radicals
- Cellular Oxygen Deficiency
- Oncogenes

- Chronic Electromagnetic Field Exposure
- Sick Building Syndrome
- Nuclear Radiation
- Pesticide/Herbicide Residues
- Chlorinated Water
- Tobacco and Smoking
- Immune-Suppressive Drugs
- Food Additives
- Dental Factors
- Diet and Nutritional Deficiencies
- Toxic Emotions
- Intestinal Toxicity and Digestive Impairment
- Viruses
- Blocked Detoxification Pathways
- Cellular Terrain
- Genetic Predisposition

weaken the body and tax its systems until they finally overwhelm the body's defenses and manifest as disease.

Sunlight—Solar radiation, particularly ultraviolet-B and ultraviolet-C radiation, is a common carcinogen, accounting for over 400,000 skin cancers of the overall one million new cases of skin cancer occurring annually in the U.S. Today, even more ultraviolet radiation is present in sunlight because the ozone hole in the Earth's upper atmosphere has expanded, weakening the Earth's natural shield against it.

Chronic Electromagnetic Field Exposure—According to an Environmental Protection Agency study, there is growing evidence of a link between exposure to electromagnetic fields (EMFs)—which are generated by electrical currents—and cancer. While EMFs are part of nature and in fact are radiated by the human body, the quality and intensity of the energy can either support or destroy health. As a rule, EMFs generated by technological devices or installations tend to be much more harmful than naturally occurring EMFs. We are surrounded by EMFs, produced by electrical wiring in homes and offices, televisions, computers, microwave ovens, overhead lights, and electrical poles. EMFs affect enzymes related to growth regulation, gene expression, and cell division and multiplication—all of which can exert a major influence on cancer tumor growth.

Geopathic Stress—Magnetic radiations from the Earth, presumably connected with geological fractures and subterranean water veins, have been associated with an increased risk of cancer in communities situated near these geopathic, or pathogenic, influences. According to some experts, the cause of geopathic stress may be localized magnetic anomalies—unusual, sudden changes and quirks that can upset delicate human physiological balance and thereby create health problems. In 1971, the theory of geopathic stress was supported by research showing that water flowing underground, especially subterranean streams that cross, produces measurable increases in magnetic anomalies; these conditions also increase electrical conductivity in the air and soil. While the changes are small, they are still capable of contributing to the development of serious illness, including cancer.

Sick Building Syndrome—In the early eighties, physicians began using the term *sick building syndrome* (SBS) to refer to a host of symptoms produced by low-grade toxic envirromnental conditions found in living, work, or office spaces. SBS symptoms are numerous: mucous membrane irritation of the eyes, nose, and throat, chest tightness, skin complaints, headaches, fatigue, lethargy, coughing, asthma, wheezing, chronic nasal stuffiness, temporary weight loss, infections, and emotional irritability. All of these depress the immune system, rendering the individual susceptible to long-term chronic illness and potentially to a cancer process. In most cases, problems with a building's engineering, construction, and ventilation system are the causes. Other sources of indoor toxic pollution include volatile organic compounds released by particleboard desks, furniture, carpets, glues, paints, office machine toners, and perfumes. In addition, the carcinogenic effects of certain indoor air pollutants, such as asbestos, environmental tobacco smoke, radon, and formaldehyde, are well described in the clinical literature and are now considered cancer risk factors.

Ionizing Radiation—Ionizing radiation consists of high-energy rays that are capable of ripping the electrons from matter, causing genetic mutations that can lead to cancer. This is the type of radiation used in X-ray technology, which may explain why radiologists (people who take many X rays each day) have historically had higher incidences of cancer, as have other workers exposed to low-dose radiation. In fact, medical X rays may cause about 75% of breast cancer. In addition to medical X rays, ionizing radiation also emanates from such common household items as fluorescent lights, computer monitors, and television screens.

Nuclear Radiation—Working or living in the proximity of nuclear power plants presents a cancer risk. Among the hazards are the small amounts of radioactive gases released daily from nuclear reactors. Although these radioactive gas emissions enter the atmosphere at levels deemed "permissible" by the U.S. Department of Energy, evidence suggests that low-level radioactive pollution may pose a significant cancer risk. In the United Kingdom, a higher rate of leukemia has been reported in children living near a nuclear facility. Finally, the incidence of childhood thyroid cancer has increased 100 times in those areas of Ukraine, Belarus, and Russia most acutely exposed to the Chernobyl nuclear accident in April 1986, according to a United Nations report. The dangers of nuclear radiation are not limited to those who work in or live close to a reactor, however. Low-level radioactive pollution returns to us in rainfall, which then accumulates in the soils to contaminate the food chain. The prime carriers for fission products were municipal water and air, and to a lesser extent, fresh milk and dairy products.

Pesticide/Herbicide Residues—Clear evidence has linked long-term exposure to pesticides with cancer, leading a consortium of 75 Environmental Protection Agency experts to rank pesticide residues among the top three environmentally derived cancer risks. Cancer-causing pesticides found in the environment and in our food tend to accumulate in fatty tissues, in fish, cattle, fowl, or people. This slow, gradual process—called bioaccumulation—will continue as long as we continue to be exposed to pesticides.

Unfortunately, the use of these poisons is not being curtailed; rather, it has increased tenfold since the introduction of DDT in the

> ## Israel Proves the Pesticide/ Cancer Link
>
> In 1978, Israel banned toxic chemicals such as DDT and PCBs which had been directly linked with breast cancer in a 1976 study.[7] Over the next ten years, the rate of breast cancer deaths in Israel declined sharply, with a 30% drop in mortality for women under 44 years old, and an 8% overall decline, despite an increase in other cancer risks such as dietary factors and alcohol consumption. Meanwhile, worldwide death rates from breast cancer had increased by 4%.[8]

1940s. In the past 50 years, some 15,000 chemical compounds and more than 35,000 different formulations have come into use as pesticides worldwide. Many of those banned in the U.S. (including DDT) are sold to Third World countries, where they enter food products, such as coffee, fruits, and vegetables, which are then imported into the U.S. In addition to agricultural pesticides, home and garden herbicides represent another major source of toxicity.

Industrial Toxins—A great number of highly toxic chemicals, materials, and heavy metals are released by industrial processes. These toxins later find their way into human tissue, where they have negative health effects, including cancer. By 1980, the Environmental Protection Agency had detected over 400 toxic chemicals in human tissue. Some industrial by-products mimic the activity of estrogen once inside the body, creating havoc in hormonal balance; these estrogen-mimicking chemicals are believed to contribute to breast cancer.

Polluted Water—Polluted water can raise the risk of developing cancer, as tap water from municipal sources is increasingly becoming a health hazard in the U.S. One out of every four public water systems has violated federal standards for tap water. It is not only pesticides and agricultural runoff that contaminate public drinking water: according to the Environmental Protection Agency, the tap water of 30 million Americans contains potentially dangerous levels of lead. Tap water can contain many different contaminants, including radioactive particles, heavy metals (such as lead and copper), radon, gasoline solvents, industrial wastes, chemical residues, disinfectant by-products, and solid particulates such as asbestos.

Chlorinated Water—Disinfecting drinking water with chlorine is standard practice throughout the U.S. While there is little doubt that adding chlorine-type compounds to drinking water protects the public from several kinds of harmful bacteria, chlorine can also form cancer-causing agents when it interacts with other compounds in drinking water. New evidence indicates that chlorinated water increases the risk of cancer for the roughly 200 million Americans who drink it.

Fluoridated Water—Fluoride, a poison second in toxicity only to arsenic, has routinely been added to public drinking water and toothpaste since the 1950s, despite mounting evidence of its multiple health hazards. According to scientific research, fluoride in drinking water can produce cancer, transforming normal human cells into cancerous ones. The National Academy of Sciences has found that fluorine (a component of fluoride) slows down DNA repair activity.

Tobacco and Smoking—About 30% of cancer deaths in the U.S. can be attributed to tobacco smoke, making it "the single most lethal carcinogen in the U.S.," according to researchers at the Harvard Center for Cancer Prevention in Cambridge, Massachusetts. Over 2,000 chemical compounds are generated by tobacco smoke, and many of them are poisons. Carbon monoxide is released during smoking, reducing the amount of oxygen to the brain, lungs, and heart. Nicotine is not only addictive, but also acts as a cancer promoter, making it easier for cancer cells of all types to spread throughout the body. Tar, the leading cancer-causing chemical found in tobacco smoke, contains carcinogenic hydrocarbons and other toxic substances.

QUICK
DEFINITION

Estrogen is one of the female "sex" hormones, produced mainly in the ovaries (some in the fat cells), that regulates the menstrual cycle. Estrogen is important for adolescent sexual development, prepares the uterus for receiving the fertilized egg by stimulating the uterine lining to grow, and affects all the body's cells; its levels decline after menopause. Estrogen slows down bone loss, which leads to osteoporosis and it can help reverse the incidence of heart attacks; estrogen also improves skin tone, reduces vaginal dryness, and can act as an antiaging factor. For the first 10 to 14 days in a woman's cycle and peaking at ovulation, the uterus is mainly under the influence of estrogen. Estrogen levels begin to climb right after menstruation, from about days 7 to 14. There are three natural types of estrogen: estradiol (produced directly from the ovary); estrone (produced from estradiol); and estriol (formed in smaller amounts in the ovary).

Hormone Therapies—Hormone therapies which increase the levels of estrogen (SEE QUICK DEFINITION) relative to progesterone in women have been linked to some forms of cancer. In particular, prolonged use of oral contraceptives and hormone replacement therapy (HRT) for postmenopausal women have been associated with an increased risk of breast and endometrial cancer. Regarding oral contraceptives, one study indicated that women who took the pill for more than four years were twice as likely as nonusers to develop breast cancer by age 50.

Immune-Suppressive Drugs—The widespread, habitual, and chronic use of a great number of conventional drugs, antibiotics, and even vaccinations can have a seriously suppressive effect on the immune system, acting in concert with all the other factors at play to prepare the system for a cancer process. Drugs such as aspirin, acetaminophen, and ibuprofen taken for aches and colds, and glucocorticosteroids such as cortisone decrease antibody production and suppress immune vitality. Antibiotics can directly hinder immune activity and increase the intestinal overgrowth of the yeast *Candida albicans*, which then can suppress the immune system. Research suggests that vaccinations can also suppress the immune system. Chemotherapy drugs used to stop cancerous growths have powerful immune-suppressive effects, rendering the individual even more susceptible to new, secondary cancers.

Irradiated Foods—The intent of food irradiation is to kill insects, bacteria, molds, and fungi and thus to extend shelf life, but the results might be dangerous to consumers. The process of irradiation leads to the formation of toxic substances, such as benzene and formaldehyde, and other toxic chemical by-products that have been associated with cancer risk. For example, food irradiation may increase the levels of aflatoxin, a deadly carcinogen; it may allow the botulinum toxin (which causes botulism food poisoning) to remain undetected in irradiated foods; over time it may induce some microorganisms to mutate, giving rise to new, dangerous species. The FDA estimates that 10% of the chemicals in irradiated foods are not found in normal (nonirradiated) foods and are unknown to science.

Food Additives—Of the 3,000 chemical additives introduced into the American food supply every year, and only a small fraction have been tested for their effects on humans (most are tested on animals). Among the most common are aspartame, saccharin, and cyclamates, artificial sweeteners that have been linked to greater incidences of cancer; butlyated hydroxytoluene, a food preservative that may contribute to liver cancer; and tannic acid, present in wines and fruits and linked to liver cancer. Other food additives that may increase the risk of certain kinds of cancer include Blue Dye No. 2, Propyl gallate, and Red Dye No. 3.

Mercury Toxicity—Mercury, a toxic heavy metal which often comprises up to 50% of "silver" dental fillings, is a noted carcinogen. Like other heavy metals, mercury has been shown to cause damage to the lining of arteries and nerve bundles, thereby contributing to cancer. In addition, heavy metals act as free radicals—highly reactive, charged particles that can cause damage to body tissues if inhaled or absorbed. The International Academy of Oral Medicine and Toxicology cites evidence indicating that dental mercury amalgams are a major contributor to immune dysfunction and free-radical pathologies, including cancer, kidney dysfunction, and cardiovascular disease.

Dental Factors—Health practitioners familiar with the principles of biological dentistry have long noted a link between dental problems and degenerative illness. When a tooth is inflamed or infected, it can block the energy flow along one or more of the body's acupuncture meridians, causing the deterioration of a corresponding organ or tissue and, in time, leading to cancer. In effect, a problem in the tooth can focus its energy imbalance elsewhere in the body, a phenomenon known as "dental focus."

Nerve Interference Fields—Dysfunctions and imbalances in the autonomic nervous system (ANS—SEE QUICK DEFINITION) can contribute to a cancer process. Most cases of chronic illness involve changes in the ANS, upsets in the electrical activity of ganglia (nerve bundles), according to Dietrich Klinghardt, M.D., Ph.D. The source of this electrical confusion is called an "interference field" or focus, and can be caused by skin scars from old accidents or surgeries; nerve bundles made toxic from an accumulation of mercury, parasite toxins, solvents, and many other substances; restriction in blood flow to the ANS from strokes or carbon monoxide poisoning; and general trauma from events such as wounds, surgical injury, or skull fracture.

QUICK
DEFINITION

The **autonomic nervous system (ANS)** can be likened to your body's automatic pilot. It keeps you alive through breathing, heart rate, and digestion, without your being aware of it or participating in its activities. The ANS has two divisions: the sympathetic, which expends body energy; and the parasympathetic, which conserves body energy. The sympathetic nervous system is associated with arousal and stress; it prepares us physically when we perceive a threat or challenge by increasing our heart rate, blood pressure, and muscle tension. The parasympathetic nervous system slows heart rate and increases intestinal and most gland activity.

Diet and Nutritional Deficiencies—According to the National Academy of Sciences, 60% of all cancers in women and 40% of all cancer in men may be due to dietary and nutritional factors. The rise of degenerative disease has paralleled the adoption of an overly refined and adulterated, high-protein, high-fat diet over the past 100 years. After World War II, the U.S. population shifted away from regular consumption of whole grains and fresh vegetables, and instead increased its consumption of less wholesome, overly refined foods. This new, so-called affluent diet is high in fat, which can more readily concentrate such chemicals as pesticides, preservatives, and industrial pollutants. High intake of animal protein, fats (especially animal fats), and refined carbohydrates and sugar is associated with an increased risk of breast cancer.

Chronic Stress—Numerous studies have linked stress and its related psychological components to susceptibility to cancer. Adults who have recently lost a loved one, or been widowed, divorced, or separated, tend to have the highest cancer rates. In addition, a basic inability to cope with stress has been regarded as a key risk factor in developing breast cancer. Unrelieved, chronic stress increases cancer risk by gradually weakening the immune system. Under emotional distress, the brain may signal the adrenal glands to produce chemicals called corticosteroids, hormones that weaken the immune response. In other words, chronic stress manifests in the body in increased adrenaline levels, hormonal changes, and decreased immune function, creating an environment in the body that may increase the risk of serious disease, including cancer.

Toxic Emotions—Since the 1970s, research in the field of psychoneuroimmunology (PNI) has documented direct links between emotions and biochemical events in the body. Noted women's health expert Christiane Northrup, M.D., of Yarmouth, Maine, coined the term *toxic emotions* to indicate the powerful, strongly held, and often unconsciously active beliefs and emotions which help generate symptoms that keep illnesses in place. In the view of Dr. Northrup as well as other alternative practitioners working with cancer patients, beliefs and emotions can be legitimate toxins, contributing to an overall weakening of the immune system.

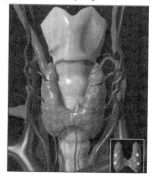

Depressed Thyroid Action—An underactive or dysfunctional thyroid gland (a key endocrine gland located in the neck) may contribute to a cancer process. Broda O. Barnes, M.D., a doctor who specialized in treating patients with hypothyroidism (underfunctioning thyroid), observed in his clinical practice evidence to suggest a relationship between low thyroid activity and cancer. Research has

The thyroid gland is the body's metabolic thermostat, controlling body temperature, energy use, and, for children, the body's growth rate.

tended to support Dr. Barnes' clinical observations. In 1954, studies by Dr. J.G.C. Spencer from Bristol, England, showed that there was a consistently higher incidence of cancer in areas of 15 countries where goiter (enlargement of the thyroid gland) was more prevalent among the population than in the non-goiter areas of the same localities.

Intestinal Toxicity and Digestive Impairment—When the intestines become clogged, toxic, and diseased by what and how we eat and by how poorly we eliminate waste material, the bowel becomes toxic. This creates toxicity for the entire body, resulting in an inability to absorb the nutrients necessary for health. Around 1900, most people in the U.S. had a brief intestinal transit time (meaning it took only about 15-20 hours from the time food entered the mouth until it was excreted as feces). Today, many people have a seriously delayed transit time of 50-70 hours—more time for stool to putrefy, for harmful microorganisms to flourish, and for toxins to develop and poison the tissues.

Mucus-producing foods such as dairy products, eggs, and meat contribute to slowing transit time. As a sticky mucoid lining builds up in the intestines as a result of eating these foods along with white flour products, it not only blocks the absorption of essential nutrients into the bloodstream but also produces a hiding place for bacteria, fungi, yeast, and parasites that are harmful to human health. An overgrowth of these organisms creates a situation called dysbiosis (an imbalance in intestinal microflora), in which the contents of the intestines putrefy and harmful chemicals are generated.

Parasites—The possible presence of parasites in the body, mostly in the intestines, is a little appreciated but major health problem. While people assume they are vulnerable to parasites only if they travel in tropical areas, the fact is that anyone can get them (and many probably already have) from merely staying at home. The damage parasites cause can be extensive: they can destroy cells faster than they can be regenerated; they can release toxins that damage tissues; and, over time, they can depress, even exhaust, the immune system. Of the dozens of specific parasites of concern to human health, the major groupings include microscopic Protozoa, roundworms, pinworms, hookworms (Nematoda), tapeworms (Cestoda), and flukes (Trematoda).

Viruses—According to some researchers, up to 15% of the world's cancer deaths are attributable to the activities of viruses, bacteria, or parasites. Among the cancer-producing viruses that work through a host's

DNA-synthesizing and protein-building mechanisms are human papilloma virus types 16 and 18 (which are sexually transmitted), associated with cervical cancer, and the hepatitis B virus, associated with liver cancer. Epstein-Barr virus, which produces mononucleosis, is also carcinogenic.

Blocked Detoxification Pathways—In a healthy individual, the body's normal detoxification systems, especially the liver, are generally able to eliminate toxins and thereby prevent illness. To prevent cancer, the liver's detoxification system must be working optimally, says Joseph Pizzorno, N.D., of Seattle, Washington. When the liver is not functioning well, it is unable to process and eliminate the multiplicity of carcinogens entering the body. "High levels of exposure to carcinogens coupled with sluggish detoxification enzymes significantly increase our susceptibility to cancer," says Dr. Pizzorno.

Free-Radical Overload—A free radical is an unstable molecule that steals an electron from another molecule, producing harmful effects. Free radicals are generated by energy production and fat metabolism, from the immune response by white blood cells, and by the liver's own detoxification process. However, uncontrolled free-radical production plays a major role in the development of at least 100 degenerative conditions, including cancer. What makes the difference between normal functioning of the immune system, which includes the deactivation of free radicals, and the initiation of cancer is the amount of antioxidants available in the system. An antioxidant (meaning "against oxidation") is a natural biochemical substance that protects living cells against damage from harmful free radicals. A negative magnetic field is a free-radical scavenger.

Cellular Oxygen Deficiency—One of the most provocative theories of cancer causation was originally put forth by two-time Nobel laureate, Dr. Otto Warburg. He was a German biochemist who won his first Nobel Prize in 1931 for the discovery that oxygen deficiency and cell fermentation are part of the cancer process. According to Dr. Warburg's theory, when cells are deprived of oxygen, they can revert to their "primitive" state, deriving energy not from oxygen, as normal cells do, but rather from the fermentation of blood sugar. Blood sugar (glucose) breaks down into lactic acid, which causes an imbalance in the body's acid/base ratio, or pH level (SEE QUICK DEFINITION); as the acidity of the body rises, it becomes even more difficult for the cells to use oxygen normally. "All normal cells have an absolute requirement for oxygen," stated Dr. Warburg, "but cancer cells can live without oxygen—a rule without any exceptions." Humans can become oxygen deficient through several routes, including long-term exposure to air pollution, devitalized foods, inadequate exercise, and maladaptive reactions.

Cellular Terrain—The term *cellular terrain*, first coined by European practitioners of what is called biological medicine, refers to the general vitality, activity, and biochemical condition of the cells in the body. When the cell becomes imbalanced, conditions are set for infection, illness, and chronic diseases such as cancer. "As we see it," explains Thomas Rau, M.D., medical director of Parcelsus Clinic in Switzerland, "sickness is not caused by bacteria, but the bacteria comes with the sickness. Bacteria, viruses, or fungi can only develop if they have the suitable cellular conditions." Outside influences, such as faulty diet, inadquate, nutrition, exposure to carcinogens, chronic free-radical toxicity, stress, or trauma provide the impetus to throw the cells out of balance, says Dr. Rau.

Oncogenes—The predominant emphasis in conventional cancer research today is to find individual genes capable of causing, initiating, or triggering cancer growth. First identified in the 1970s, these causal genes are referred to as oncogenes (meaning the gene that starts the *onkos*, or tumor mass). Oncogenes are believed to transform normal cells into cancer cells. Researchers now believe that about 20% of all human cancers are partly brought about by oncogene mutations. In healthy people, the activities of oncogenes are counterbalanced by tumor suppressor genes, also called antioncogenes. Under normal conditions, these genes act to prevent uncontrolled cell growth that could lead to tumors.

Genetic Predisposition—The theory of gene causation for cancer inevitably leads researchers into speculations about inherited cancers—genetic configurations or mutations that might predict if not guarantee that a given individual will develop a particular form of cancer. The term *family cancer syndrome* is now used to describe the tendency of particular cancers (such as breast, colon, or ovarian) to show up in succeeding generations of the same family. Many scientists now believe that the following inherited cancers may be linked to mutations in certain related tumor suppressor genes: melanoma and pancreatic cancer (MTS1, p16); breast and ovarian cancer (BRCA1); breast cancer (BRCA2); colon and uterine cancer (MSH2, MLH1, PMS1, PMS2); and brain sarcomas (p53).

Why Cancer Grows

While these predisposing factors may be important, cancer only develops under certain conditions within the human body, no matter what genetically damaging carcinogens may be involved in the initiation of the disease. The two most important conditions that must exist for the development of cancer are acidity and the lack of oxygen; that is, the pH of the cellular environment must be acid and there must also be a deficiency of oxygen in the cells where cancer is growing. These two conditions are collectively known as acid-hypoxia.

As mentioned above, Otto Warburg was given a Nobel Prize for demonstrating that acid-hypoxia is necessary for cancer to develop and grow. Other researchers since his initial discovery have confirmed his findings.[9] However, this factor in the development of cancer has been ignored by conventional medicine. The opposite condition of acid-hypoxia is alkaline-hyperoxia, when the pH of the cellular environment is alkaline and there is an optimum level of oxygen present. Cancer cells cannot live in an alkaline-hyperoxia environment.

The fuel on which the body's cells run is called adenosine triphosphate (ATP—SEE QUICK DEFINITION). ATP must be created by all cells, including cancer cells, for energy. The biochemical process in which ATP is created is called oxidation phosphorylation and is oxygen-dependent. Healthy cells require the conditions of alkalinity and high molecular oxygen (O_2) to produce ATP and function properly. In contrast, non-oxygen-respiratory organisms—like cancer cells—make ATP by fermentation phosphorylation, which requires the conditions of acidity and low oxygen to function, and actually produces additional acids. The most common acid produced is lactic acid.

DEFINITION

ATP stands for adenosine triphosphate, a substance found in all cells, particularly muscle, and responsible for energy. When enzymes split ATP, energy is released from the high-energy phosphate bonds. This bond can be instantly split on demand whenever energy is required to run cellular functions. Then ATP becomes ADP. When energy is returned, it becomes ATP again. ATP is often called the cell's energy currency because it can be continually spent and remade again in a matter of minutes.

When cells are deprived of oxygen, they enter into fermentation reactions, deriving energy not from oxygen but rather from the fermentation of glucose. For example, when we exercise vigorously and use up our energy and oxygen supplies, muscle cells will temporarily resort to fermentation phosphorylation to produce ATP. However, since we are oxygen-dependent respiratory organisms, fermentation cannot continue to properly sustain cellular life for a long period of time.

The oxidation of normal cells and fermentation processes of cancer cells work under directly opposite and conflicting conditions. These two mechanisms of making energy directly oppose each other and are totally incompatible. As we will see, magnetic therapy can help alkalinize and oxygenate tissues, thus removing the conditions necessary for cancer cells to survive.

Success Story: Basal Cell Carcinoma

Suzanne, 71, had suffered a sunburned forehead several years ago. Every now and then, a basal cell carcinoma (skin cancer) would appear on her forehead as a result of this intense sunburn. Before magnets were available to her, she would have this cancerous growth surgically removed. This time, when the skin cancer reappeared, it was successfully treated with a negative magnetic field.

This area was small enough to use a 1" x $^1/_4$" neodymium disc magnet. Every night, Suzanne slept with this magnet fastened, negative side down, directly over the cancerous area. In six weeks, the cancer dried up and peeled off without a scar. She then continued to sleep with magnets at the crown of her head, and the rough, scaly area, which had periodically become cancerous, cleared up completely. Five years later, the cancer has not returned.

In addition, magnetic field therapy can reduce the side effects of chemotherapy. For example, Mark had been treated with chemotherapy for his cancer prior to using magnet therapy. Two years later, as the cancer was still present, Mark's oncologist advised a second course of chemotherapy. During his first chemotherapy treatment, Mark had lost his hair, fingernails, and toenails; during the second course, he did not lose them. The oncologist asked Mark what he had done differently this time. Mark told him he was sleeping on a negative-poled magnetic bed pad. It may be that the entrance of magnetic therapy into oncology will be furthered by this example, in which a patient's exposure to a negative magnetic field reduced the harsh side effects of chemotherapy.

Success Story: Cancer of the Liver and Spleen

Don, a physician/anesthesiologist, had a rapidly expanding abdomen and increasing weakness. Oncologists determined that he had cancer of the liver and spleen, and that these two organs were so full of cancer that they were causing swelling in his abdomen. He was deemed a hopeless case, as no conventional treatment could help him. In searching for other options, he discovered magnet therapy and learned how to treat himself. He placed a 4" x 6" x $\frac{1}{2}$" ceramic magnet over his spleen and another one over his liver; the swelling in both of these organs gradually receded. Don decided to continue to treat himself because he is a knowledgeable physician. As it turned out, his magnetic treatment protocol was completely successful. There is now no evidence of cancer in his liver or spleen.

Success Story: Prostate Cancer

Thomas was diagnosed as having prostate cancer with bone metastases (cancer that has spread to the bone). He was treated by placing a 4" x 6" x $\frac{1}{2}$" ceramic magnet on his lower abdominal area with the negative magnetic field facing the body. He did this whenever sitting down, about 3-4 hours a day. He also permanently fastened a flexible 4" x 12" x $\frac{1}{8}$" magnet across his sacral area (near the tailbone). Three months later, X rays revealed no evidence of bone cancer, and the PSA (prostate specific antigen, a cancer marker for prostate cancer) had dropped from an initial 28 to 2, which is within the normal limits.

Success Story: Malignant Melanoma

Roberta, 75, suddenly developed a fast-growing, invasive mole on her forehead. The mole was black and red, with jagged edges and a very sore base. In one week, it grew to be one inch across and half an inch high. It had also penetrated into the subcutaneous fat and had the clinical appearance of a serious, malignant melanoma.

She elected to try magnetic therapy. In her first week, she was treated during her sleep with a neodymium disc magnet. Unfortunately, this 1" x $\frac{1}{4}$" magnet was slightly smaller than the surface of her melanoma tumor, so the mole continued to grow, its edge becoming wider and more notched. Obviously, the magnetic field needed to be larger than this lesion and the duration of exposure also needed to be longer. She was then exposed 24 hours a day to a $1\frac{1}{2}$" x $\frac{1}{2}$" ceramic disc magnet. With continuous negative magnetic field exposure, the tumor stopped growing and its soreness eased after one month. Then the tumor started to recede and dry up. After ten weeks, it literally fell off her forehead.

Success Story: Malignant Brain Tumor

Michael, 20, was diagnosed with an inoperable malignant glioblastoma, a type of brain tumor. He was left unconscious and unresponsive to environmental stimuli. The negative magnetic field from a 4" x 6" x $\frac{1}{2}$" ceramic magnet was placed on the back of his head where the tumor had started growing, and was continued 24 hours a day.

Three days later, his consciousness returned and he was able to wiggle his fingers and respond to questions. In three weeks, he walked out of the hospital with only the assistance of a walker. He continued the treatment on his brain for an extended period of time. After this dramatic turnaround, he has remained well for the past five years, and his tumor has not returned.

Treatment Options for Cancer

The incompatibility of oxidation and fermentation for making energy is important for treating cancer. Quite simply stated, oxidation phosphorylation protects us because it blocks fermentation phosphorylation. The human bio-oxidative energy system is capable of defeating the biological energy system of cancer cells. Since cancer cells are non-oxygen-respiratory biological cells, they die in an oxygen-rich and alkaline environment. So, if enough oxygen is made available in an alkaline cellular environment, this inhibits the possibility of cancer cells growing, reproducing, and thriving within the body.

≥CAUTION≥

Cancer patients should not treat themselves without the guidance of a physician who understands magnetic therapy.

Magnet Therapy

When a negative magnetic field is applied to the body, it has the ability to remove the cancer-developing condition of acid-hypoxia and replaces it with an alkaline and oxygenated environment. Therefore, a negative magnetic field exposure can be used to treat as well as prevent cancer. A negative magnetic field (supplied internally, applied externally, or both) treats cancer in the following ways:

■ A negative magnetic field creates an alkaline environment for all cells, tissues, and organs exposed to the field. In doing so, it acts directly on the bicarbonate buffer system to maintain a normal and healthy tissue state.

■ A negative magnetic field serves as an energy activator for the oxidoreductase enzyme system, which effectively processes and eliminates free radicals (including peroxides, acids, alcohols, and aldehydes). It releases oxygen (O_2) from its bound state in these harmful products and further oxygenates the body.

A negative magnetic field exposure creates bodily conditions in which cancer cannot exist. This oxygen-rich and highly alkaline environment inhibits the energy-making functions of cancer cells. Because of this fact, a negative magnetic field of sufficient strength and duration can cause the death of cancer cells.

A continuous and sufficiently high gauss exposure of a negative magnetic field to a cancerous lesion reverses cancer, irrespective of the type of cancer. My observations are that the cancer cells exposed to a continuous and sufficiently high-gauss negative magnetic field do not revert back to normal cells—instead, they die.

In addition, tumors that are still present after magnetic treatment have been microscopically examined and found to be no longer neoplastic (subject to abnormal growth). If the tumor is a surface lesion (such as a melanoma), then new skin will grow under the tumor and it will eventually fall off.

The acid-hypoxic condition associated with cancer cells always produces swollen cells, or edema. When cells become swollen, then DNA cellular repair does not occur, mutations develop, and cells lose their ability for normal metabolism. This leads to the further proliferation of cancer cells. Negative magnetic field exposure can reduce edema, so that DNA injuries can be healed. If treated with a negative magnetic field before mutation occurs, edema can be reduced and injured cells can be returned to normal functioning cells.

The negative magnetic field is the essential energy source that governs the normal healing process in general. Robert O. Becker, M.D., demonstrated that a negative magnetic field is the necessary element for any form of healing to occur.[10] During the healing process, the body concentrates a negative magnetic field at the site of injury to initiate and sustain healing. An external negative magnetic field produces the same healing effects.

Clinical studies show that a negative magnetic field reduces the cellular division and growth of cancer cells and a positive magnetic field increases this growth.[11] In one study, researchers exposed cancer cells to a negative magnetic field. After three weeks, the negative magnetic field produced a significant decrease in cancer cell growth. They also observed that the positive magnetic field produced a small, but detectable, increase in cancer growth. Other studies confirmed that a static magnetic field inhibits the growth of three human tumor cell lines *in vitro*[12] and produced positive results in women with breast cancer.[13]

Using Magnets for Cancer Therapy

Cancer is a serious disease, so one must treat it with an optimum level of magnetic energy. The first principle of cancer treatment is to provide a solid baseline of systemic treatment, by sleeping on a magnetic bed pad along with magnets at the crown of the head. The magnets in the bed pad are 1⁷/₈" x ⁷/₈" x ³/₈" mini-block magnets, placed 1¹/₂" apart throughout the pad.

The magnets at the crown of the head are held firmly up against the headboard in a wooden carrier. This carrier contains four 4" x 6" x 1" ceramic magnets placed ³/₄" apart, which can be raised or lowered depending upon the height of the pillow. This provides a magnetic field of 19" x 6"; a person can turn from side to side and still be within this field. In addition, the top of the head should be as close to the magnets as possible.

To treat metastatic cancer systemically, use a super magnetic bed (70 4" x 6" x 1" ceramic block magnets placed 1" apart). Sleep on this bed through the night and for four 1-hour periods during the day; treatment should last at least three months. Breast cancer should be considered as systemic, even if there are no known metastases.

In maintaining health and reversing degenerative disease, it is important to have deep, energy-restoring sleep. The depth of sleep is controlled by the hormone melatonin, made during sleep by the pineal gland in the center of the brain. This gland generates melatonin in response to a negative magnetic field. Accordingly, you should magnetically treat the head during sleep, in order to raise melatonin levels.

Furthermore, the retina of the eyes as well as the intestinal wall produce melatonin. The eyes can be treated at night with a magnetic eye unit, composed of a magnetic light shield with 1" x ¹/₈" neodymium disc over each eye.

If possible, the cancer patient should also sleep with a 5" x 12" double magnet, multi-magnet flexible mat across the lower abdomen. Also, a 4" x 6" x ¹/₂" ceramic magnet should be placed lengthwise on the body in the center of this mat (held in place with a 4" x 52" body wrap). This treatment will stimulate the wall of the gastrointestinal tract to produce melatonin.

Whenever sitting down during the day, sit on a chair pad containing 1⁷/₈" x ⁷/₈" x ³/₈" mini-block magnets, placed 1¹/₂" apart throughout the seat and back. Also, place a 4" x 6" x ¹/₂" ceramic magnet under the seat, back far enough to radiate into the genital area.

Rules for Magnetic Treatment of Cancer

Cancer may be a local lesion or have multiple metastases. It is effective and fairly simple to treat a single cancerous lesion that is not interfering with such basic functions as the gastrointestinal tract, the lungs, or liver function. Each lesion must be treated separately with a magnetic field that is larger than the lesion. Metastatic cancer needs to be treated systemically.

The following rules apply to the local treatment of cancer:

■ Always use the negative magnetic field.

■ The magnetic field must be larger than the lesion being treated.

■ The magnet must have close proximity to the lesion being treated, preferably directly over the lesion.

■ A minimum of 25 gauss must reach the cancer.

■ Treatment must be continuous or as continuous as possible. The only exceptions to continuous treatment are brief breaks to take a bath or allow for digestion after meals.

■ The minimal time required to treat cancer is 12 weeks. Since magnetic treatment is not harmful or symptom-producing, it is safe to extend it beyond this time. Slow-growing cancers, such as basal cell carcinoma, have been reversed by treating only at night during sleep. However, fast-growing cancers, such as malignant melanoma, require exposure 24 hours a day.

■ Treating at right angles is permissible. In other words, place a magnet directly over the organ and another at a right angle to the organ.

■ When treating internal organs, use larger and stronger magnets in order to achieve more penetration. These magnets include the 4" x 6" x $1/2$" or 4" x 6" x 1" ceramic magnets.

■ If the lesion is raised, as in the case of a melanoma, then use a cushion or a pad so as not to put pressure on the lesion. The neodymium disc magnet is ideal for treating melanomas that are less than an inch across. Use the ceramic disc magnet if the melanomas are less than $1^1/_2$" across. Spread the magnetic field by first placing a 2" x 2" or 3" x 3" plastiform magnet on the lesion and then a neodymium disc magnet on top. If the melanomas are larger than this, then a larger magnet must be used.

Wear a magnet over the heart during the day, since this will magnetize the water and oxygen flowing through the heart. Use a 5" x 6" double magnet, multi-magnet flexible mat, held in place by pinning it to the clothing. If possible, place this magnet between the inner and outer clothing, with two 1" x $1/8$" neodymium disc magnets placed on the outer clothing to hold the mat in place. The multi-magnet flexible mats have been designed to fit around the curved surfaces of the body, such as the breasts or joints. The magnetic field can be spread and reinforced by placing a ceramic or neodymium magnet on top of the mat.

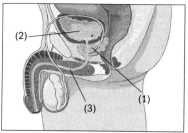

The prostate (1), a male sex gland, is located below the bladder (2) and encompasses the urethra (3).

Clearly, these magnetic therapies may be somewhat cumbersome and uncomfortable at times. The person attempting them, however, must remember that the effectiveness of the magnetic therapy is dependent on increasing the strength and duration of the magnetic exposure. Obviously, therefore, day and night magnetic exposure is the best procedure when attempting to kill cancer cells within the body.

Prostate Cancer–Always use a negative magnetic field, negative pole side facing the body. For local treatment, sit on a chair pad (containing 1⅞" x ⅞" x ⅜" magnets placed 1½" apart throughout the seat and back of the pad) with a 4" x 6" x ½" ceramic magnet under the pad directly beneath the genital-rectal area. The more hours of treatment, the better the results.

For systemic treatment, use a magnetic bed pad (containing 1⅞" x ⅞" x ⅜" magnets, placed ½" apart). Place a 5" x 12" double magnet, multi-magnet flexible mat crosswise on the lower abdomen. In the center of this, place a 4" x 6" x ½" ceramic magnet lengthwise. This can be held in place with a body band. Also use four magnets (6" x 4" x 1") at the crown of the head, placed ¾" apart in a wooden carrier on the headboard. The holder can be raised or lowered depending on the height of the pillow. The magnets should be at the level of the back of the head and as close as possible to the top of the head.

Cancer of the Lips and Mouth–Always use a negative magnetic field, negative pole side facing the body. Place a 5" x 6" multi-magnet flexible mat across the mouth to cover the lips, chin, and the area between the upper lip and the nose. Place a 4" x 6" x ½" ceramic magnet on each side of the face, extending sufficiently forward for the magnetic field to cover the nose. This local treatment should be kept in place continuously, except for the brief periods of washing or eating. The minimum duration is three months. Systemic treatment is optional (see Prostate Cancer, above).

Malignant Melanoma–Always use a negative magnetic field, negative pole side facing the body. Tape a cushion (with a hole in the middle, as those used for bunions) over the malignant mole to prevent pressure on it; use hypoallergenic tape. Tape a 1" x $^1/_8$" super-neodymium disc magnet on the cushion. The magnet needs to be larger than the lesion being treated. For systemic treatment, see Prostate Cancer above.

In addition, sleep with magnets on the front and back of the chest. Use a 5" x 12" x $^1/_8$" double magnet, multi-magnet flexible mat held in place with a body wrap supported by shoulder straps. This magnetizes the oxygen in the lungs, which then circulates throughout the body and prevents the spread of cancer. During waking hours, wear a 5" x 6" double magnet, multi-magnet flexible mat over the heart with the negative pole facing the heart. Eliminating a malignant melanoma may take three to four months of treatment.

Breast Cancer—This protocol deals with only a single lesion in the breast that has not metastasized to the lymph tissue or bones. It applies equally to treating either a primary lesion or the area of post-surgical (or post-chemotherapy) removal.

Use a 5" x 12" double magnet, multi-magnet flexible mat and place directly over the affected breast. The mat can be held in place with either a bra or a 4" x 52" body wrap with shoulder straps. Place a 1$^1/_2$" x $^1/_2$" ceramic disc directly over the lesion or area where surgery has been done.

Science Demonstrates the Power of Magnetic Therapy

The French Academy of Sciences published a report in March 1965, on the magnetic treatment of mice with lymphosarcoma. Every mouse in the untreated or control group died within 15 to 18 days. In three other groups, mice began magnetic treatment at different points in time, but with the same strength and duration of magnetic treatment: 620 gauss for two hours a day.

The first group received magnetic treatment within five days of starting the test and recovered quickly; all tumors and metastases disappeared. The second group began treatment on day seven and showed the same recovery as the first group; a third group of mice was treated from the tenth day on, but did not recover. These mice all died in 19 to 22 days, just after the untreated mice had died.[14]

These findings were compelling enough to encourage the French Academy of Sciences to conduct another experiment, this time testing the effect of the daily dosage given. In the first group, the mice were treated from the fifth day, with 620 gauss one hour a day; in the second group, the mice were treated with 620 gauss two hours a day, also from the fifth day. Once again, the results were striking. As expected, all the mice in the untreated (control) group died within 15 days; all the mice in the first test group died after 19 days. Meanwhile, the mice in the second test group—they received twice the magnetic treatment per day as the first group—all survived and showed no signs of cancer.[15]

Magnetizing Oxygen and Water

For all forms of cancer, perhaps the most ideal systemic treatment is to magnetize the oxygen that is being breathed. This is achieved by using an oxygen concentrator. Expose the oxygen concentrator's tubing to the negative magnetic field of a 4" x 6" x 1" ceramic magnet "oxygen magnetizer." Usually, this oxygen magnetizer is used at night during sleep.

This type of treatment needs to be continuous in order to achieve magnetized oxygen's effect. If continuous treatment cannot be maintained, then treat all night while asleep, as well as in one-hour increments three or four times during the day. It is ideal to combine local cancer treatment with breathing magnetized oxygen.

Water also is magnetizable. Whenever a part of the body is treated with a magnetic field, the water in the body within that field is being magnetized. In addition, drinking water can be magnetized by simply placing it on the negative field side of a ceramic magnet. The water will be magnetized within five minutes of exposure.

Although this disc will magnetically adhere to the mat, you may want to tape it in place. If the lesion is larger than $1\frac{1}{2}$", then place a 4" x 6" x $\frac{1}{2}$" ceramic magnet over the area.

Whenever possible, use the 11" x 17" multi-purpose pad, placed on top of the magnets that are already on the breast. At night, it should be used on the abdomen and also across the breast. Whenever sitting down, sit on the magnetic chair pad that has magnets in the seat and back; the more hours of exposure, the better.

Breast cancer is a systemic disease, even if there is no known metastatic spread. During sleep or while resting during the day, lie down on the magnetic mattress pad and sleep with magnets at the crown of the head. The best systemic treatment is the 70-magnet bed, composed of 4" x 6" x 1" magnets placed 1" apart.

Pelvic/Colon Cancer—This protocol is suitable for cancers in the low abdomen area, including the prostate, cervix, vagina, uterus, and colon. Place a 5" x 12" double magnet, multi-magnet flexible mat crosswise on the lower abdominal area. Directly over the center of this mat, place a 4" x 6" x $\frac{1}{2}$" ceramic magnet lengthwise on the body. Hold these magnets in place with a 4" x 52" body wrap. Maintain this placement 24 hours a day for at least three months and preferably longer.

Whenever sitting down, sit on the chair pad that has magnets in the seat and back. Place a 4" x 6" x $\frac{1}{2}$" ceramic magnet under the seat far back enough to radiate into the genital area. When convenient, place the 11" x 17" multipurpose pad over the lower and upper parts of the abdomen. This pad should also be used over the abdominal area during sleep. The more hours of exposure to the chair pad and multi-purpose pad, the better. At night, sleep on the magnetic mattress pad and place magnets in the carrier against the headboard. Also, sleep with a magnetic eye unit across the face.

Place a 5" x 12" double magnet, multi-magnet flexible mat over the heart and chest, held in place with a 4" x 52" body wrap around the chest. The wrap should be loose enough to allow normal breathing. Keep this magnetic mat in place 24 hours per day to magnetize the oxygen and water passing through the heart. The flow of negative magnetized oxygen and water throughout the entire body will help to maintain an optimum pH as well as discourage the spread of cancer.

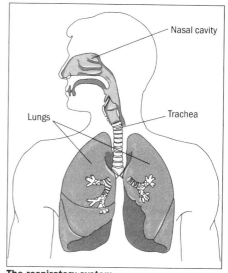

The respiratory system.

Lung Cancer—Place a 5" x 12" double magnet, multi-magnet flexible mat across the chest and another across the back; hold these mats in place with a 4" x 52" body wrap. Furthermore, place a 4" x 6" x $1/2$" ceramic magnet directly over the lesion. The body wrap around the chest should be loose enough so there are no restrictions while breathing. The magnets should be kept on the chest 24 hours per day. This also applies to the 4" x 6" x $1/2$" ceramic magnet placed over the lesion. Exposure should be maintained for at least three months, but preferably four months or more.

Whenever sitting down, sit on a magnetic chair pad. Also, place the 11" x 17" multipurpose pad over the abdomen and pull it up over the chest so it is on top of the other magnets. Lung cancer should also be treated systemically using the 70-magnet bed system. During sleep or while resting during the day, lie down on a magnetic mattress pad and sleep with magnets at the crown of the head. Also, one should stimulate melatonin production by using the previously described magnetic therapy. Obviously, when treating any form of cancer, the more hours of exposure, the better.

For the **Four-Day Diversified Rotation Diet**, see Appendix.

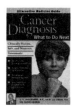

For more **alternative medicine treatment options for cancer**, see *Cancer Diagnosis: What to Do Next* (Alternative Medicine.com Books, 2000; ISBN 1-887299-40-8); to order, call 800-333-HEAL.

Other Treatment Considerations

The majority of cancer patients have various maladaptive reactions to foods, such as allergic, addictive, or toxic reactions. So, cancer patients should follow a Four-Day Diversified Rotation Diet to improve the function of the immune system and help the fight against cancer. Nutrition should also be optimized—testing for deficiencies of specific vitamins, minerals, trace elements, amino acids, essential fatty acids, hormones, and digestive enzymes should be done by a knowledgeable physician and treated accordingly. The cancer patient should also avoid tobacco, alcohol, caffeine, food additives, perfumes, or any addictive substances. Exposure to toxic chemicals in the home and workplace should be kept to a minimum.

There are, of course, methods that reduce the risk factors involved in the development of all forms of cancer. These methods include:

1) Avoidance of tobacco

2) Avoidance of alcohol

3) Limiting exposure to home and industrial chemicals, pesticides, poisons, perfumes containing potentially carcinogenic chemicals, and air pollution

4) Getting optimum exercise

5) Improving nutrition, which includes the optimum intake of vitamins, minerals, amino acids, fiber, and essential fatty acids, and also the low intake of fat and sugar, as well as the complete avoidance of all chemical food additives

6) Prevention of sunburn or prolonged exposure to the sun

7) Eliminating allergic and addictive reactions to all foods, chemicals, and inhalants

Children's Health Problems

NATURAL AND ALTERNATIVE approaches such as magnet therapy can be very effective in maintaining a child's health, as well as treating common childhood illnesses with no harmful side effects. Certain standard medical treatments such as the extensive use of antibiotics and immunizations are being challenged by researchers, physicians, and government officials with regard to their safety and overall effectiveness.

Caring for children is a demanding and sometimes difficult task for parents. When sickness arises, parents may feel frustrated by not being able to identify what is wrong with the child, as well as in not being able to determine the severity of the condition. When dealing with a childhood illness, parents need to evaluate the condition of the child and decide what steps to take. Today, physicians and parents have many options in caring for children, especially in the area of alternative medical care.

Bed-Wetting

Involuntary wetting of the bed (enuresis) in the middle of night is common during childhood, but usually spontaneously stops by the teenage years. Bed-wetting in children beyond the age of normal bowel training is often caused by maladaptive reactions to foods and chemicals. Other potential underlying causes include hypoglycemia, diabetes, urinary tract infections, emotional stress, small and weak bladders that cannot hold the urine all night, excessive consumption of liquids, and behavioral problems.

Treatment Options for Bed-Wetting

A Four-Day Diversified Rotation Diet should be used as a primary

For the **Four-Day Diversified Rotation Diet**, see Appendix.

treatment for this condition. Nutritional supplements that may be helpful for bed-wetting include:

- Mixed amino acid supplements (two capsules, 2-3 times daily, ten minutes before meals)
- Magnesium (100 mg two times daily)
- Calcium (250 mg with dinner and before bed)
- Vitamin B complex (one tablet with breakfast and lunch)
- Multivitamin (two to three daily)

One should also closely examine the child's living environment and eliminate any potentially harmful chemical exposure. Allergies can be a major cause of bed-wetting; reactions to foods or environmental factors can cause sudden and violent contractions in the muscles of the bladder.

Also, the child should sleep on a magnetic bed pad and with four 4" x 6" x 1" ceramic magnets at the crown of the head. Improving sleep with magnetic treatment will help reduce the child's bed-wetting problem.

Behavioral Disorders

Children's behavioral disorders include hyperactivity, hostility, aggressiveness, learning disorders, and attention deficit. Hyperactivity is a complicated and often misunderstood condition. It has been categorized with conditions such as hyperkinetic syndrome, minimal brain dysfunction, and attention deficit disorder (ADD). A child who is inattentive, overly talkative, impulsive, excessively irritable, and is hyperactive is labeled as ADD.

Hyperactivity may be caused by a learning disability, an unstable home life, food allergies, food addiction, food additives, heavy metal toxicity, or even the need for glasses. Health practitioners often find that many ADD patients improve when taken off sweeteners such as sugar and corn syrup. A recent study performed at Yale University School of Medicine provided a possible reason as to why sugar induces hyperactive reactions in some children. The investigation revealed that, when ingested by children, sugar releases twice the amount of the stimulant hormone adrenaline into the bloodstream, as it does in adults.[1]

Viral infections, such as Epstein-Barr, cytomegalo, or human herpes virus #6, are another potential underlying cause. These types of infections may be acquired either during gestation or in early childhood. They degrade the proper functioning of both the immune system (B lymphocytes) as well as the neurons in the brain (neurons in

CHILDREN'S HEALTH PROBLEMS

the pre-frontal, frontal, and temporal areas of the brain are especially affected).

Treatment Options for Behavioral Disorders

The immediate symptoms of these disorders are often reduced by bitemporal placement of either the 1½" x ½" ceramic disc magnets or 1" x ⅛" neodymium disc magnets. Place these magnets near the top of the front of the ears and hold in place under a sweatband or a 2" x 26" self-fastening band. Sitting on a comfort chair pad, which has magnets in the seat and in the back, is often helpful in these disorders.

For the **Four-Day Diversified Rotation Diet**, see Appendix.

It is extremely important to follow a Four-Day Diversified Rotation Diet as well as implement an optimum nutritional support program. Eliminating sugar from the diet does not by itself solve the problem. Glucose is not the problem—rather, it's an addiction to foods from which sugar is derived. Often, environmental factors can exaggerate a condition such as hyperactivity.

Caffeine, found in many brands of soda pop, is another culprit in children's behavioral disorders and should be reduced or eliminated. In a survey involving 800 school children, those consuming sodas containing caffeine were more likely to be labeled as hyperactive by their teachers than those who drank caffeine-free soda.[2]

Approximately 5,000 food additives are used in food products in the United States.[3] Benjamin Feingold, M.D., conducted extensive research on the possible link between attention deficit disorder, food additives, and naturally occurring salicylates and phenolic compounds. Studies have both supported[4] and dismissed[5] this theory. However, the National Institutes of Health Consensus Development Conference on Defined Diets and Childhood Hyperactivity had decided that further investigation into the role food additives may play in ADD is warranted.[6] Most recently, a joint project between German and British researchers has suggested that food intolerance or allergies may contribute to hyperactivity.[7]

Chronic Fatigue Syndrome

WHEN THE FIRST CASES of chronic fatigue syndrome (CFS) were identified in the 1980s among patients in a small Nevada town, the strange disease—marked principally by deep fatigue and muscle aches—was dubbed "Yuppie flu." It seemed to be concentrated among young, affluent white professionals. Due to this and to the subjective nature of the symptoms, CFS was the butt of jokes and its sufferers were often not taken seriously, even by many physicians. CFS has now become an epidemic and crossed all ethnic and demographic barriers. It is now recognized as a severe, debilitating illness, although the previously dismissive attitude persists in some doctors.

The U.S. Centers for Disease Control (CDC) reports that 80% of diagnosed cases are women, the majority of whom are white and between the ages of 25 and 45. However, these figures reflect underreporting among nonwhite populations.[1] Meanwhile, the number of chronic fatigue cases continues to rise. The CDC offers a typically conservative estimate of four to ten cases per 100,000 adults,[2] but other sources place the numbers much higher.

According to Murray R. Susser, M.D., of Santa Monica, California, chronic fatigue syndrome (also known as chronic fatigue and immune dysfunction syndrome, CFIDS) afflicts an estimated three million Americans and 90 million people worldwide. Jesse A. Stoff, M.D., co-author of *Chronic Fatigue Syndrome: The Hidden Epidemic*, believes it is even more widespread, estimating that the number of people with CFS in North America alone exceeds by four million the number of people with AIDS.[3]

Chronic fatigue syndrome (and fibromyalgia) is a syndrome that is accompanied by a cluster of symptoms that seem to develop

Symptoms of Chronic Fatigue Syndrome and Fibromyalgia

Allergies	Increased thirst	Poor concentration
Anxiety	Irritability	Prolonged fatigue
Brain fog and confusion	Joint and muscle pain	after exertion
Cough	Low body temperature	Rashes
Decreased appetite	Low-grade fever	Recurring infections
Depression	Memory loss	Severe fatigue
Digestive disorders	Muscle weakness	Sleep problems
Dizziness	Nausea	Sore throat
Dry eyes and mouth	Night sweats	Swollen lymph nodes
General stiffness	PMS (women)	Visual blurring
Headaches		

together rather suddenly. These symptoms can include: deep fatigue unrelieved by sleep, muscle and joint pain or weakness, headache, memory loss, mental confusion and poor concentration, digestive problems, recurring infections, low grade fever (often in the afternoon), swollen lymph glands, food and environmental allergies and sensitivities, severe exhaustion from minor activity, and depression.

Other possible symptoms associated with CFS include dizziness, anxiety attacks, night sweats, rashes, breathing irregularities, irregular heartbeat, and hypersensitivity to heat and cold and to light and sound. The degree and severity of these symptoms often fluctuate, not only over a period of weeks or months, but even from day to day.

What Causes Chronic Fatigue?

There is no single cause of chronic fatigue syndrome; rather, multiple factors combine to overwhelm the immune system and produce the breakdown known as CFS. Prominent among these factors are: concurrent infections, such as Epstein-Barr virus (EBV), the cytomegalo virus, and the human herpes virus #6; candidiasis (yeast overgrowth); an underactive thyroid gland; stress and adrenal exhaustion; toxic overload; nutritional deficiencies; allergies; and extensive use of antibiotics, hydrocortisone, or vaccinations.[4]

My clinical experience indicates that CFS and fibromyalgia stem from the above viral infections combined with maladaptive (and addictive) food reactions.

Multiple Factors That Contribute to CFS

- Multiple infections—viruses, bacteria (such as *Borrelia burgorferi*, the cause of Lyme disease), candidiasis, parasites
- Immune dysfunction
- Thyroid and hormonal problems
- Mercury toxicity
- Enzyme deficiencies
- Allergies
- Food addictions
- Nutritional deficiencies
- Lifestyle issues—stress, psychological/emotional factors

Treatment Options for CFS

Nutritional deficiencies are often a feature of chronic fatigue syndrome. As with most of the factors involved in this disorder, it is difficult to tell which came first, the deficiencies or the immune breakdown. The immune and other physiological systems of the body need proper nutrients in order to maintain health. Without enough or the right kinds of nutrients, these systems cannot operate at an optimum level. If the nutritional deficiency becomes chronic, breakdowns in function will occur.

In addition, a body whose immune system is continually overactive, as it is in CFS, requires far more nutrients to keep it going than a healthy body does. Conversely, this overactive immune system with its accompanying nutritional drain can in itself lead to deficiencies in key nutrients.

Those with CFS should first have a careful nutritional evaluation, including a complete examination of levels of vitamins, minerals, trace elements, amino acids, hormones, and essential fatty acids. Vitamin B12, for example, deserves special attention, since a B12 deficiency makes people weak. Vegetarians are especially prone to vitamin B12 deficiency.

Diet

The Four-Day Diversified Rotation Diet is essential for all those with CFS. Maladaptive reactions to foods are a common complaint of people who suffer from chronic fatigue syndrome. Allergies and the immune response they generate can be an underlying factor in up to 80% of patients with chronic fatigue.[6] As a contributor to immune overload, ongoing allergic reaction is an essential condition to address in the treatment of CFS. Maladaptive reactions to any substance (foods, chemicals, or inhalants) can produce CFS. It is imperative to first identify these substances and then avoid them. In addition, one should avoid the use of caffeine, tobacco, and alcohol.

For the **Four-Day Diversified Rotation Diet**, see Appendix.

Diagnosing CFS and Its Causes

G etting a clear picture of an individual's CFS is often difficult due to the tendency of symptoms to fluctuate in degree and severity, not only over a period of weeks or months, but even from day to day. A cyclical pattern of illness and reasonable health is the result. Frequently, after a severe bout of CFS, a patient resumes normal activity and exercise, only to relapse into extreme fatigue after a period of time. But if a number of CFS symptoms persist for six months and other causes have been eliminated, it is considered likely that the person has CFS.[5]

Without determining precisely what is happening in the patient's body, treatment is guesswork. A careful medical history, a physical examination, and selected laboratory tests can pinpoint the imbalances, deficiencies, infectious agents, and specific immune system weaknesses which are contributing to your CFS and provide the physician with an inventory of the pattern of symptoms. Most of the testing involves simple blood, urine, and stool analyses, but your conventional doctor may not be aware of the specific parameters to investigate.

Eliminate Infections

Viruses, candidiasis, bacterial infections, or intestinal parasites (SEE QUICK DEFINITION) are often a factor in chronic fatigue syndrome. Whether these infections in combination are the cause of CFS or opportunistic invaders of an already weakened immune system has not been conclusively determined. In either case, infections involved perpetuate and deepen immune dysfunction by further taxing an already overloaded system. One infection puts demand on the immune system which can't kick it, and another infection may join in, leading from one to another in a domino effect. The most common infections are yeast and parasites. Hidden bacterial infections such as Lyme disease and abscesses in the teeth and sometimes chronic sinusitis and gastritis may also be factors.

The damage caused by parasites in particular can be quite extensive. Parasites can destroy cells faster than they can be regenerated; they can release toxins that damage tissues, resulting in pain and inflammation; and, over time, they can depress, even exhaust, the immune system.

Magnetic therapy can help to eliminate any infections related to CFS. As discussed in the chapter on infections, a negative magnetic field can eliminate infectious microorganisms of all kinds from the

QUICK
DEFINITION

A **parasite** is any organism that lives off another organism (called a host), and draws nourishment from it. Specifically, parasites are the protozoa (single-cell organisms), arthropods (insects), and worms that infect the body and cause serious damage to tissues and organs. Common forms of the protozoan parasites are *Giardia lamblia*, which causes giardiasis; *Entamoeba histolytica*, which causes dysentery; and *Cryptosporidium*, which causes diarrhea, particularly in people with immunologic diseases such as AIDS. The most common arthropod parasites are lice, mites, ticks, and fleas. Worm parasites include pinworms, roundworms, tapeworms, whipworms, *Trichinella spiralis* (worms usually acquired from eating tainted pork), hookworms, Guinea worms, and filaria (threadlike worms that inhabit the blood and tissues).

Testing for Nutritional Deficiencies

Unfortunately, a person with CFS is likely to be receiving fewer nutrients than someone who is healthy. This is because the various viruses, parasites, fungal overgrowths, and other infections characteristic of CFS are draining nutrients from the person suffering from the disorder. In addition, with gastrointestinal disorders, such as candidiasis and the "leaky gut" syndrome which can result, many of the nutrients from food and even supplements are not being absorbed by the body.

As with other aspects of treatment, in order to design an effective program of nutritional supplementation, it is necessary to identify all deficiencies. Thorough testing can avoid prescribing the wrong supplement and save time and expense in the long term. Among the laboratory tests for nutrient status, the four discussed below are relatively inexpensive and provide detailed, practical information.

Individualized Optimal Nutrition (ION)—Using a blood and a urine sample, the ION (Individualized Optimal Nutrition) Panel from MetaMetrix measures 150 biochemical components. The test is highly useful for physicians who need detailed biochemical assessment of patients who have chronic fatigue or other immune disorders, multiple chemical sensitivities, cancer, heart disease, learning difficulties, or obesity. Specifically, ION checks for nutritional status in categories including vitamins, minerals, amino acids, fatty and organic acids, lipid peroxides, general blood chemistries (cholesterol, thyroid hormone, glucose), and antioxi-

dants. In each category, a patient's levels are compared with predetermined limits.

FIA™ (Functional Intracellular Analysis)—These tests (as Comprehensive Profile 3000, B-Complex Profile 1100, Primary Profile 1500, Cardiovascular Profile 1600, or Antioxidants Profile 1400) measure the function of key vitamins, minerals, antioxidants, amino acids, fatty acids, and metabolites (choline, inositol) at the cellular level. They also assess the status of carbohydrate metabolism in terms of insulin function and fructose intolerance.

Pantox Antioxidant Profile™—Using a small blood sample, this diagnostic screen measures the status of more than 20 nutritional factors as a way of determining the body's antioxidant defense system. It then compares the results against a database of 7,000 normal and healthy profiles. Specifically, the screen reports on

For **ION**, contact: MetaMetrix Medical Laboratory, 5000 Peachtree Industrial Blvd., Suite 110, Norcross, GA 30071; tel: 770-446-5483 or 800-221-4640; fax: 770-441-2237. For **Functional Intracellular Analysis™**, contact: SpectraCell Laboratories, Inc., 515 Post Oak Blvd., Suite 830, Houston, TX 77027; tel: 713-621-3101 or 800-227-5227; fax: 713-621-3234; website: http://www.spectracell.com. The **Pantox Antioxidant Profile** must be ordered by a licensed health-care practitioner. Contact: Pantox Laboratories, 4622 Santa Fe Street, San Diego, CA 92109; tel: 888-726-8698, 619-272-3885 or 800-726-8696; fax: 619-272-1621. **Oxidative Protection Screen** must also be ordered by a licensed health-care practitioner. Contact: Antibody Assay Laboratories, 1715 East Wilshire #715, Santa Ana, CA 92705; tel: 714-972-9979 or 800-522-2611; fax: 714-543-2034.

body. In this regard, the negative magnetic field acts like an antibiotic. Systemic treatment should be used for infections. Sleep on the 70-magnet bed, using 4" x 6" x 1" magnets placed 1" apart, every night and for four 1-hour periods during the day, for a minimum of three months.

Boost Energy

Energy-draining physical and mental symptoms associated with CFS can be treated with a negative magnetic field. In particular, applying a 5" x 6" multi-magnet flexible mat over the heart magnetizes the oxygen and water flowing through the entire body, producing a systemic healing effect that helps CFS sufferers.

For additional systemic healing at night, sleep on a magnetic bed pad. This pad is composed of mini-block magnets ($1^7/_8$" x $^7/_8$" x $^3/_8$") placed $1^1/_2$" apart. At the crown of the head, there should be a carrier holding four magnets up against the headboard; these are 4" x 6" x 1" ceramic magnets placed $^3/_4$" apart. The top of the head should be as close as possible to these magnets.

Applying a negative magnetic field to the head and body during sleep increases the production of melatonin and growth hormone. These two hormones govern the entire energy system of the body.

Hormones

Thyroid problems, particularly an underactive thyroid gland (hypothyroidism), are often implicated in chronic fatigue syndrome. While hypothyroidism is technically considered a separate illness and not a cause of CFS, many CFS patients have not been properly tested

For more about **magnet therapy and infections**, see Infections.

for thyroid problems and distinct categorization of the two illnesses is not necessarily of benefit to the patient. Eliminating or confirming the thyroid as a factor should be a first step in the investigation of what is causing your CFS.

Hormonal imbalances are also common in CFS; specifically, imbalances or deficiencies in the adrenal hormones DHEA (SEE QUICK DEFINITION) and cortisol and the hormone ACTH (adrenocorticotropic hormone, secreted by the pituitary gland). Since the adrenal glands play a central role in maintaining the body's energy levels, when these glands are functioning poorly, the result is fatigue. Low amounts of melatonin, the pineal gland hormone that regulates the body's sleep cycle, may also be contributing to the overall symptom picture of CFS.

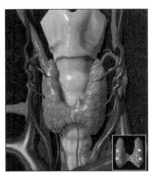

The **thyroid gland**, one of the body's seven endocrine glands, is located just below the larynx in the throat, with interconnecting lobes on either side of the trachea. The thyroid is the body's metabolic thermostat, controlling body temperature, energy use, and, for children, the body's growth rate. The thyroid controls the rate at which organs function and the speed with which the body uses food; it affects the operation of all body processes and organs. Of the hormones synthesized in and released by the thyroid, T3 (tri-iodothyronine), represents 7%, and T4 (thyroxine), accounts for almost 93% of the thyroid's hormones active in all of the body's processes. Iodine is essential to forming normal amounts of thyroxine. The secretion of both these hormones is regulated by thyroid-stimulating hormone, or TSH, secreted by the pituitary gland in the brain.

In the case of hypothyroidism, clinical studies reveal that many subjects need to reduce or totally eliminate thyroid supplementation once magnetic therapy increases their melatonin production. However, if magnet therapy does not work, then the patient's thyroid function should be examined. Several other primary causes may be involved with thyroid malfunction and may need to be treated with thyroid supplementation.

For adrenal insufficiency, a correction of this disorder will often occur as a result of the negative magnetic field's power to raise melatonin levels in the body. Melatonin controls the function of both the thyroid and adrenal hormones. An adequate production of melatonin can often serve to correct hypothyroidism and adrenal insufficiency, both of which are associated with chronic fatigue.

However, adrenal cortical hormones may be required as supplements. The positive magnetic field can also stimulate the production of adrenal hormones. This method consists of placing the positive magnetic field from a 4" x 6" x $\frac{1}{2}$" magnet over the adrenal area (atop the kidneys) for a period of only three to five minutes. There is no reason to extend exposure beyond this time, as the optimum production of adrenal hormones will occur within this short period. This should be done upon awakening in the morning.

Alleviating Depression

Everyone with chronic fatigue and fibromyalgia does not have the same psychological or emotional makeup, but all have a psychological component to their illness. As a result, unless stressful lifestyle practices and the emotional factors contributing to your illness are thoroughly addressed, no cure will ever be complete and lasting.

During the day, depression can be treated with bitemporal placement of $1^1/_2$" x $^1/_2$" ceramic disc magnets or 1" x $^1/_8$" super neodymium disc magnets. Symptoms will often improve in 10-30 minutes. For relief of anxiety, place a disc magnet on the forehead and another on the left temporal area. For relief of obsessive-compulsiveness, place a disc magnet on the left temporal and another on the low occipital (base of the skull) area. Whenever sitting down, use a comfort chair pad, with mini-block magnets in the seat and back (magnets are $1^7/_8$" x $^7/_8$" x $^3/_8$"). Also, place a 4" x 6" x $^1/_2$" ceramic magnet under the seat of this comfort chair pad as far back as the genital area.

DEFINITION

DHEA (dehydroepiandrosterone) is naturally produced by the human adrenal glands and gonads with optimal levels occurring around age 20 for women and age 25 for men. After those ages, DHEA levels gradually decline so that a person 80 years old produces only a fraction of the DHEA they did when they were 20. As an antioxidant, hormone regulator, and the building block from which estrogen and testosterone are produced, DHEA is vital to health. Low DHEA levels have been associated with cancer, diabetes, multiple sclerosis, hypertension, obesity, AIDS, heart disease, Alzheimer's, and immune dysfunction illnesses. Test subjects using supplemental DHEA reported improved sleeping patterns, better memory, an improved ability to cope with stress, decreased joint pain, increases in lean muscle, and decreases in body fat.

Diabetes

ACCORDING TO THE U.S. Department of Health and Human Services, nearly 6 million people in the United States suffer from diabetes, which is now the seventh leading cause of death among Americans. *Diabetes mellitus* is a term used to describe the condition characterized by various reactive and seesaw fluctuations in blood sugar (glucose) and insulin levels. In most cases, the hypoglycemic (low blood sugar) and hyperglycemic (high blood sugar) states that characterize diabetes both have the same basic source of allergy/addiction. In fact, it is now apparent that abnormally high or low blood sugar levels in the body are caused for the most part by maladaptive allergic reactions to specific foods of all types, chemicals, and inhalants.

Whether the body's response to these substances is low or high blood sugar depends on the stage of the stress reaction. Analogous to Hans Selye's general adaptation syndrome (GAS) for stress, hypoglycemia can be considered the adaptation stage of the stress allergic reaction, and hyperglycemia, which is diabetes mellitus, can be considered the exhaustion stage. Both of these medical conditions are manifestations of an underlying degenerative disease process. The central factor of this disease process is the chronic maladaptive reactions to specific foods, chemicals, and inhalants as addictive stressors. These chronic addictive stressors clearly disorder and exhaust all biochemical metabolic processes.

There are two major types of diabetes mellitus. These are Type I insulin-dependent juvenile diabetes and Type II non-insulin-dependent adult-onset diabetes.

Type I diabetes mellitus usually begins in childhood, but it may occur at any time in life if the pancreas is damaged due to chronic IgG immunologic and non-immunologic maladaptive food reactions, chronic viral infections, injury, or disease. Up to 10% of those diagnosed with diabetes are Type I diabetics.

In Type I diabetes, the body is unable to produce adequate insulin. As a result, glucose builds up in the bloodstream and spills over into the urine. The body "starves to death" because the cells cannot get enough nourishment, normally supplied by glucose, to produce energy and/or to carry out their normal functions. Symptoms of Type I diabetes include excessive thirst, hunger, urination, dehydration, and weight loss. The insulin injection is currently the only method to control Type I diabetes mellitus. This treatment, however, is not considered a cure.

Most diabetics have Type II diabetes, which usually occurs in middle age. Symptoms are the same as for Type I, with the exception of weight loss. In Type II diabetes, the pancreas still produces insulin, but the body cells are resistant to its action and therefore cannot absorb the glucose produced by food intake. This phenomenon is referred to as insulin resistance. Insulin resistance is a manifestation of cellular edema from maladaptive reactions to foods and chemicals.

Type II diabetes mellitus is a reversible disease.[1] The statistics supporting the reversal of the disease process have been gathered on Type II diabetes, but there are no such statistics on Type I diabetes. However, there is good reason to believe that early and appropriate treatment of viral infections, IgG food reactions, and addictions to foods, chemicals, and inhalants can prevent the progression of the disease process to insulin dependence. In addition to withdrawing from all foods, chemicals and inhalants to which one might maladaptively react, one must also control all viral, fungal, and bacterial infections as well as maintain an optimum nutritional environment.

Either type of diabetes, when poorly controlled, can lead to heart and kidney disease, atherosclerosis, hypertension, strokes, cataracts, retinal hemorrhages, neuropathy (nerve damage), gastroparesis (loss of peristaltic action in the gastrointestinal tract), gangrenous infections of cuts or sores (with possible amputation of the feet or legs), loss of hearing, blindness, and even death. These complications are easier to avoid in both types of diabetics if blood sugar levels are kept as close to the normal range as possible.

What Causes Diabetes?

Although a genetic predisposition appears to govern susceptibility to both types of diabetes, a number of other factors can also be involved.

Diet and obesity are key elements in the cause of Type II diabetes. Autoimmune processes, in which antibodies created to fight allergies or viral infections react against the body itself, may also play a role in causing both types of diabetes.

Type I Diabetes

In Type I diabetes, the insulin-producing cells of the pancreas have been destroyed and are unable to produce any more insulin. Seventy-five percent of Type I diabetics have antibodies to their own pancreatic cells, as opposed to 0.5% to 2.0% of individuals without diabetes, supporting the theory of an autoimmune cause of the disease.[2] Viral infections are often implicated as initiating the immune and autoimmune disease process associated in Type I diabetes. These viral infections usually proceed by direct inflammatory infection of pancreatic beta cells. The most likely viruses implicated include pertussis, hepatitis, rubella, Coxsackie, Epstein-Barr, cytomegalo, and human herpes #6. Milk allergy may be a factor in initiating autoimmune reactions in Type I diabetes.

Type II Diabetes

Food addiction is the cause of Type II diabetes. Diet, obesity, addictions and allergies to certain foods, viral infections, and stress are all factors that can contribute to the onset of or aggravate Type II diabetes. The main cause of obesity is a food addiction, and the key factor is not how much but what is consumed.

The insulin resistance (a state in which glucose does not properly enter cells, resulting in hyperglycemia or high blood sugar levels) observed in Type II diabetics is caused by a chain reaction of metabolic events. Maladaptive reactions to foods, chemicals, and inhalants are the initial cause in this series of undesirable metabolic events. These reactions produce acidity and a deficiency of oxygen in cells and tissues. As a result, these reactions cause edema or swelling of cells throughout the body. In addition, if the maladaptive reactions are chronic, then nutritional and enzyme deficiencies begin to develop, which further exacerbate the diabetes disease process.

It is important to understand that insulin resistance is separate from, and not dependent on, the amount of insulin present. Initially, the Type II diabetic has enough insulin, but it cannot do its job properly in acid-hypoxic cells. Later in the disease process, the pancreatic cells also become acid-hypoxic and reduce their insulin production. However, this reduced amount of insulin is secondary to the maladaptive reactions. The failure to isolate the major cause of insulin resistance is the fundamental error in the conventional diagnosis and treatment of Type II diabetes.

Success Story: Diabetic Neuropathy

Nerve deterioration may occur in any part of the body as a complication of diabetes. Pain is the most common symptom in diabetic neuropathy, with the arms, shoulders, neck, legs, or feet typically involved. Placing a negative magnetic field over the painful area is the most effective treatment, superior to the usual conventional drug treatment (with nonsteroidal, anti-inflammatory agents). Magnetic therapy will often relieve the pain where none of these usual pain-relieving agents is successful.

John had diabetic neuropathy and experienced severe, burning pain in the soles of his feet. He had found no relief with conventional pain medications. Placing both of his feet on the negative pole of four ceramic magnets (4" x 6" x ½") relieved his pain within a few minutes and he remained pain free for several hours. Each time the pain in his feet returned, John repeated this magnetic treatment. After the magnets had consistently relieved his pain over six treatments, the pain ceased, and the magnets were no longer needed.

Success Story: Gangrene

The skin of diabetics is not healthy and quite commonly, especially in the feet, ulcers will develop. These ulcers will most often be of a mixed type of bacterial and fungal infections, which may produce gangrene. The local area of infection can be treated with a negative magnetic field.

Frank, 74, had gangrene of his right foot. As a result, he was undergoing EDTA chelation (SEE QUICK DEFINITION). Unfortunately, the chelation treatments were not helping his severe problem; in fact, he was scheduled to have the gangrenous foot surgically removed. About a week before the operation, Frank placed the negative pole of a 4" x 6" x ½" ceramic magnet to the sole of his infected foot. Within one week of continuous exposure, the improvement was so substantial that his foot was not amputated. Within a month of treatment, the gangrenous foot had healed.

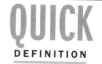

DEFINITION

Chelation therapy refers to a method of binding up ("chelating") toxins (e.g., heavy metals) and metabolic wastes and removing them from the body while at the same time increasing blood flow and removing arterial plaque. One type of chelation therapy involves the chelating agent disodium EDTA given as an intravenous infusion over a 3½ hour period. Usually 20 to 30 treatments are administered at the rate of one to three sessions per week.

Treatment Options for Diabetes

Insulin resistance reverses and diabetes disappears when the acid-hypoxic metabolic process that creates swollen and poorly functioning cells is stopped. The primary way to stop this disease process is to strictly avoid the foods, chemicals, and inhalants that initiate symptoms. As insulin resistance begins to disappear, the requirement for an external source of insulin is lowered dramatically. I have clinically observed that only one-third of the amount of insulin is necessary once a patient treats the food reactions and addictions that can be avoided on a Four-Day Diversified Rotation Diet. Some diabetics who have completely eliminated their food reactions and maintained an individually determined, optimum nutritional program have been able to totally eliminate their insulin injections.

For the **Four-Day Diversified Rotation Diet**, see Appendix.

Eighty percent of Type II diabetics are obese at the time of diagnosis. Obesity is caused by food addictions and compulsive overeating. After five days of fasting, the hyperglycemia is present only to addictive foods. Treating these addictions by rotating foods will allow weight reduction to occur and alleviate the food addictions leading to diabetes.

The program for Type II diabetics includes an initial five days of eating foods seldom consumed by the subject, followed by four weeks of test meals of single foods, including monitoring for symptoms and for blood sugar changes before and after the meal. Treatment consists of the rotation diet that leaves out the offending food for three months, followed by the gradual addition of these foods back into the rotation diet. Due to the danger of complications, food testing cannot be carried out with Type I diabetics, so their food sensitivities need to be determined by other hypersensitive testing. Most diabetics, both Type I and Type II, cannot tolerate cow's milk.

Nutrients

Diabetes should primarily be managed using the Four-Day Diversified Rotation Diet. Diabetic patients should correct any nutritional deficiencies with supplements. They should have a qualified physician arrange for testing and, if possible, offer nutritional advice. A number of nutrients have proven valuable in treating diabetes:

B Vitamins: Levels of vitamin B6 in the body drop sharply after the age of 50, when Type II diabetes is most likely to occur.[4] Vitamin B6 taken daily can reduce insulin needs and improve basic health.[5] Type II

Addictions, Allergies, and Diabetes

Conventional allergists test IgE reactions, which make the person immediately ill, but ignore, to a great degree, delayed IgG reactions, as well as the pH changes during these IgG reactions. In essence, therefore, they have ignored the foundational building blocks of the diabetic disease process. The recent documentation that IgG milk allergy is involved in Type I diabetes should encourage physicians to look much more closely at the application of allergic avoidance in diabetes.[3]

In addition, there needs to be new research regarding diabetes and the following areas:
1) IgG food reactions
2) Non-immunologic food addictions and maladaptive chemical and inhalant reactions
3) Addiction to tobacco, alcohol, and caffeine
4) The role of infections
5) The role of nutritional deficiencies
6) The role of pH
7) The role of the negative magnetic field

My experience in diagnosing and treating Type II diabetes shows that most of these cases are reversible if you start treatment early. Even in the late phase, some relief can be achieved, giving the person a more comfortable lifestyle. And even though we cannot reverse insulin need in Type I diabetes, we can do much to control it so that the deteriorated stage does not develop.

diabetics regained normal blood sugar levels with doses of 100 mg daily of vitamin B6 in tests by John Ellis, M.D., who recommends 50 mg daily for maintenance.[6] Symptoms of diabetic neuropathy were reduced or totally eliminated by vitamin B6 supplements in clinical studies.[7]

Biotin, a component of the vitamin B complex, works synergistically with insulin and helps in glucose utilization.[8] Research has shown that biotin is also beneficial for preventing and managing peripheral neuropathy in diabetics.[9] Diabetic neuropathy also responds well to vitamin B12 when it is used in conjunction with topical application of capsicum, a cayenne pepper extract that relieves the pain of neuropathy. Capsicum works by removing substance P, a pain mediator, from the skin. Niacinamide (vitamin B3) can be very beneficial in the early stages of Type I diabetes.

Vitamin C: A high intake of vitamin C has been found to reduce insulin needs, maintain eye health, and help prevent cataracts.[10] It is also important in helping to fight infections, to which diabetics are particularly prone. Megadoses of vitamin C have also been shown to prevent or delay the vascular complications of diabetes by promoting the production of collagen, which strengthens the blood vessels. However, renal (kidney) function should be tested first because megadoses of vitamin C can be toxic in a diabetic with renal insufficiency. A deficiency of vitamin C has been shown to cause degeneration of the insulin-producing cells of the pancreas.[11]

Vitamin E: According to Evan Shute, M.D., co-founder of Canada's Shute Foundation for Medical Research, vitamin E is essential for the treatment of diabetes.[12] Vitamin E is a powerful antioxidant, and has a significant anticlotting effect which may be a factor in preventing premature atherosclerosis and the development of vascular complications such as damage to the eyes and kidneys seen frequently in diabetes.[13] Supplementation of vitamin E has freed some Type II diabetics from taking insulin, and has also been shown to reduce the rate of blood clotting in Type II diabetes.[14]

Chromium: The body's chromium stores are mobilized immediately when either glucose or insulin enters the bloodstream. Even the slightest deficiency of chromium upsets the body's tolerance to glucose. The lack of chromium in the modern American diet is acute[15] and is aggravated by consumption of refined sugar, which robs the body of stored chromium.[16] Chromium supplements are effective in treating hypoglycemia (low blood sugar) and act as a "normalizer" of glucose for insulin-dependent diabetics.[17] Exercise appears to increase the levels of chromium in the tissues and increases the number of insulin receptors on cells in Type I diabetics.[18] Chromium has been shown to restore normal insulin function in Type II diabetics.[19] In a group of Type II diabetics, normal glucose tolerance was restored by 50% with daily doses of 150 mcg of trivalent chromium (the only type of chromium believed to be biologically active in the human body).[20]

Magnesium and Potassium: Deficiencies of magnesium and potassium create a greater glucose intolerance and contribute to damage to organs and the nerves that supply them due to disturbed cell function.[21] Magnesium is essential for the maintenance of a healthy cardiovascular system as well.[22] It reduces plasma lipids (fats in the bloodstream) and serum cholesterol (cholesterol circulating in the blood), is an effective vasodilator (used to widen blood vessels), and helps prevent retinopathy and atherosclerosis. Diabetics who have experienced ketoacidosis are particularly likely to be magnesium deficient. Insulin administration also induces hypokalemia (low blood potassium levels), while potassium supplementation helps improve insulin sensitivity, responsiveness, and secretion.[23]

Zinc: Zinc is essential for the normal production of insulin and the digestion of proteins,[24] and has antiviral effects. To confirm a need, ask a doctor for a white blood cell or saliva test.

Coenzyme Q10: Coenzyme Q10 stimulates production of

insulin.[25] Andrew Weil, M.D., suggests taking 80 mg a day for at least three months to stabilize blood sugar levels.[26]

Amino Acids: These assure the body's supply of raw materials for manufacture of insulin, which is composed of 51 amino acids.[27]

Digestive Enzymes: The use of pepsin and the digestive enzymes protease, amylase, and lipase is sometimes recommended to aid in the digestion and absorption of nutrients, especially in cases of diabetes where the pancreas is not functioning optimally.[28]

Magnet Therapy

For those who cannot totally eliminate their insulin injections with a Four-Day Diversified Rotation Diet and nutritional supplementation, proper magnetic treatment will aid in reducing insulin requirements, insulin resistance, and the fundamental causes involved in Type I and Type II diabetes. Magnetic therapy is a significant aid in preventing and reversing the maladaptive food reactions that ultimately cause diabetes. In addition, magnetic therapy is extremely valuable in treating many of the secondary cardiovascular complications.[29]

For more about **magnet therapy for heart disease**, see Heart Disease.

The negative magnetic field has the power to dramatically reverse most if not all of the maladaptive reactions by quickly and dramatically activating the oxidoreductase enzymes as well as increasing the oxygen and the alkaline levels in the body. The negative magnetic field also reduces edema, acidity, pain, infections, wounds,[30] and other disordered metabolic functions associated with diabetes.

All diabetics should sleep on a magnetic mattress pad that provides a full negative magnetic field exposure. In addition, sleep with magnets in a wood carrier containing four 4" x 6" x 1" ceramic magnets, placed against the headboard of the bed. Also helpful is an eye unit composed of a magnetic light shield over both eyes and much of the face. Place one or two 1" by 1/8" neodymium disc magnets over each eye, attached to the magnetic eye unit.

It is important to magnetically treat the entire body, because any cellular or tissue swelling from maladaptive reactions is corrected by a negative magnetic field exposure. As a result, insulin begins to work as it should in transporting blood sugar into the cells of the body and insulin resistance disappears.

Environmental Illness

ENVIRONMENTAL ILLNESS is a multiple-symptom, debilitating, chronic disorder involving prolonged, heightened, and often incapacitating allergies or sensitivities to numerous common substances found in one's environment. Symptoms may include headaches, fatigue, muscle pain and/or weakness, coughing or wheezing, asthma, weight loss, infections, and emotional fluctuations, depression, and/or irritability. The illness is sometimes referred to as "20th-century disease" because patients become allergic to and functionally incompatible with many products and substances found in the modern world, such as car exhaust, synthetic carpets, plywood and other building materials, cleaning agents, office machines, and plastics, among others.

Another source of problems is electromagnetic fields (EMFs) in the environment. An electromagnetic field can be likened to an invisible energy web (shaped somewhat like the contour lines on a topographical map) that is produced by electricity that in turn creates a magnetic field. While EMFs are part of Nature and in fact are radiated by the human body and its individual organs, the quality and intensity (called respectively frequency and gauss field strength) of the energy informing this contoured web can either support or destroy health. As a general rule, EMFs generated by technological devices tend to be much more harmful than naturally occurring EMFs.

Particularly harmful are the pulsing frequencies of an AC current, the type of current commonly found in households. A frequency above 12 cycles per second is stressful to humans—an AC current is 60 cycles per second. Seldom is the magnetic field associated with these currents high enough to cause stress; rather, it is the intensity of the pulsing field that is essentially harmful and the accompanying positive magnetic field of an AC current. The negative magnetic field is not stressful.

Researchers once thought EMFs, especially the very low frequency and extremely low frequency kind, were safe because they were of such low strength compared to other forms of radiation, such as those from a nuclear reactor or X rays, for example. But now, as technology grows and proliferates and people are using more and more electronic devices, some researchers suspect EMFs are contributing to a subtle assault on people's immune systems and sense of well-being.

Electromagnetic changes in the environment can adversely affect the energy balance of the human organism and contribute to disease. We are surrounded by stress-producing, electromagnetic fields generated by the electrical wiring in homes and offices, televisions, computers and video terminals, microwave ovens, overhead lights, electrical poles, and motors that can generate higher than naturally occurring pulsing frequencies. EMFs interact with living systems, affecting enzymes related to growth regulation, pineal gland metabolism (regulation of the sleep hormone, melatonin), and cell division and multiplication.

What Causes Environmental Illness?

We are exposed to toxins every day of our lives, in chemicals and pesticide residues, mercury amalgam dental fillings, biological contaminants such as pollen and parasites, and genetically altered foods, among other sources. Even our own bodies can produce toxins, called endobiotics, which can prove harmful to us if not properly controlled.

Toxins in the Environment

Toxins emanate from a variety of noxious sources, but chiefly from environmental pollution. Unavoidably, many of us carry around an internal "chemical cocktail" derived from absorbing industrial by-products (coal tar or fuel exhaust), pesticides, herbicides, household contaminants (found in cleaners, paints, plastics, and solvents), and biological contaminants (pollens, molds, dust mites, and parasites). We are also exposed to toxins from processed or genetically altered foods, alcohol or tap water (which usually contains heavy metals), and even the newspaper (from the inks used in printing).

Since the 1980s, physicians began using the term *sick building syndrome* (SBS) to refer to a host of symptoms produced by low-grade toxic environmental conditions found in living or office spaces. SBS symptoms include respiratory, eye, and skin diseases, headaches, memory loss, fatigue, lethargy, temporary weight loss, infections, irritability, and impaired balance. All of these suppress the immune system, rendering the individual suceptible to long-term chronic illness.

Office workers are exposed to toxic air that is continuously recycled throughout sealed buildings. According to William Lee Cowden, M.D., a clinical researcher in Richardson Texas, the air inside most modern buildings is five to 100 times more toxic than the outside air.[1] Since most people in industrialized nations spend more than 90% of the time indoors, these indoor concentrations of pollutants can lead to a permanent chronic exposure to toxic factors. This hazard received national publicity when CBS's *60 Minutes* disclosed that the head office of the Environmental Protection Agency in Washington, D.C., has been proven to be environmentally unsafe for its workers. In most cases, problems with a building's engineering, construction, and ventilation system are the causes. Add to this the toxic vapors and fumes produced by construction materials and bio-electromagnetic pollution, and the result is new, seemingly inexplicable illnesses that affect neurological and biochemical processes.

Xenobiotics or environmental estrogens (SEE QUICK DEFINITION) have been linked to endocrine disruption and to severe breakdown of the integrity of the digestive system, which can lead to arthritis.[2] Each year, an estimated 1,000 new synthetic chemicals enter the world market, swelling the planetary total to well over 100,000. All of these are completely foreign and potentially harmful to the function of the digestive system and endocrine glands (SEE QUICK DEFINITION). Evidence is accumulating that these chemicals, even at very low concentrations and exposures, cause "hormone havoc"—autoimmune diseases, clinical depression, and reproductive system disorders, among others.

Toxins can also enter the body in ways other than through breathing or swallowing—in particular, through the skin's pores. (Those same pores, of course, also facilitate the elimination of toxic chemicals). Approximately 70% of the toxins from tap water enter the body through the skin; the remaining 20% of the toxins enter via ingestion. Tap water in the United States contains chlorine, aluminum, pesticides, lead, copper, and other toxic substances.[3]

QUICK DEFINITION

Environmental estrogens are foreign compounds and/or chemical toxins that mimic the effects of estrogen in the body. Environmental estrogens, also called xenobiotics or xenoestrogens, are present primarily in man-made chemicals ("greenhouse gases," herbicides, and pesticides such as DDT) and industrial by-products (from manufacture of plastics and paper, as well as from the incineration of hazardous wastes).

Endocrine glands, including the testicles, ovaries, pancreas, adrenals, thyroid, parathyroid, and pituitary, are central to the regulation and normalization of all the body's complex, interconnected systems, from metabolism and heat production to spermatogenesis and uterine preparations for pregnancy.

Harmful Metals and Chemicals

Conventional dental amalgams or "silver" fillings are actually made of tin, copper, silver, nickel, zinc, and the toxic metal mercury. These fillings disintegrate over time, and have been shown in some instances to release these toxic metals into the body, affecting the bones, the joints, and the central nervous system and brain. Evidence now shows that mercury amalgams are the major source of mercury exposure for the general public, at rates six times higher than those found in fish and seafood.[4] Mercury and other toxic metals increase free radicals, which attack cell membranes and initiate swelling and inflammation.

Copper-lined pipes in plumbing systems can be another source of toxicity. A greenish-brown ring around the tub, sink, or toilet can indicate that your water is contaminated with copper, which is toxic at high levels. Extremely high levels can have a destructive effect upon protein structures, such as joint cartilage. According to Paul C. Eck, Ph.D., and Larry Wilson, M.D., of Phoenix, Arizona, many of the most prevalent metabolic dysfunctions of our time are in some way related to a copper imbalance and/or copper toxicity. Copper toxicity can cause liver problems, adrenal fatigue, allergies, and osteoarthritis.[5] Individuals who drink unfiltered water, as well as welders, metal and construction workers, plumbers, and auto mechanics can be exposed to potentially toxic levels of copper. Other sources of copper include birth control pills and intrauterine devices, and many fungicides and pesticides—all of which contain copper as a main ingredient. A thorough analysis from a health-care practitioner, including nutritional and heavy-metal assessment, can determine whether copper detoxification or supplementation is needed.

Chemicals found in dry-cleaning fluids (trichloroethylene), paint solvents (toluene), municipal water supplies (phenol and chlorine), carpets and flooring (formaldehyde), and some imported produce (DDT pesticide residues) are also potentially harmful, depending on your level of susceptibility. Studies have proven that these chemicals can interfere with proper nerve and muscle function, cause skeletal and muscular changes, and alter mental functioning.[6]

Sources of EMFs

The greatest concern about EMFs is not from a one-time use of a hair dryer or an hour on a computer, but from cumulative exposures: hour after hour, day after day, continuous high levels of EMFs. For example, people who travel extensively in airplanes can have high exposure rates, up to 85 milligauss in the airplane cabin. The EMF exposure from hair dryers, heaters, electric shavers, and other appliances can be injurious to health over time. Food mixers, hair dryers, and vacuum cleaners emit EMFs that are 30 to 100 times greater than the suggested safe limit of the pulsing field.[7] Ordinary household appliances tend to generate larger cumulative EMF exposures than power lines. The reason is proximity: most people do not live close enough to power lines to be greatly affected by their EMFs, but the situation is different with kitchen appliances, computers, cellular phones, televisions, even electrical outlets if they're located behind the head of a bed. Although the EMFs from appliances drop off at a distance of about 16 feet, people often stand or sit closer than this to the source of EMFs—typically 18 inches from computers, a few feet from televisions, and almost no distance from cellular phones.[8]

Another concentrated source of EMFs is the fuse box where the electric power line branches off from the neighborhood utility pole to your house. That fuse box—which connects the outside line with the inside wiring—generates large amounts of EMFs on a continual basis. EMFs are able to penetrate through normal building walls, but they decrease in force dramatically as you move further away from the generating source. Another potential EMF source is the wiring in your home. Older wiring sometimes generates high amounts of EMFs at the electrical outlets where you plug in your appliances.

Outside the home, electric power lines can also be a major EMF source. Some scientists allege that exposure to electric and magnetic fields generated by electric power lines is reponsible for certain cancers, reproductive dysfunction, birth defects, neurological disorders, and Alzheimer's disease. Some activist groups believe the hazard to be so great that they are calling for closure of schools and other public facilities near power lines and restructuring of the entire electric power delivery system.[9] Dr. Becker says we are constantly exposed to a background level of EMFs generated by the electric power delivery system. In urban areas, this so-called ambient field level, which is inside and outside the home, could exceed three milligauss. In the suburbs, the ambient or surrounding field ranges from 1-3 milligauss. Dr. Wertheimer and others said in their studies on power lines that constant surrounding levels of three milligauss or more were significantly related to increases in the risk of childhood cancer. Dr. Becker advocates one milligauss as a safe limit for continuous exposure to 60-hertz fields (the usual kind generated by electric power systems).[10]

Inside the Sick Building Syndrome

In the early 1980s, physicians began using the term *sick building syndrome* (SBS) to refer to a host of symptoms produced by low-grade toxic environmental conditions found in living, work, or office spaces. SBS symptoms are numerous: mucous membrane irritation of the eyes, nose, and throat, chest tightness, skin complaints (dryness, itching, abnormal redness), headaches, fatigue, lethargy, coughing, asthma, wheezing, chronic nasal stuffiness, temporary weight loss, infections, and emotional irritability. All of these depress the immune system, rendering the individual susceptible to long-term chronic illness.

"Indoor air pollution in residences, offices, schools, and other buildings is widely recognized as a serious environmental risk to human health," explains Michael Hodgson, M.D., M.P.H., of the School of Medicine at the University of Connecticut Health Center in Farmington. Dr. Hodgson notes that most people in industrialized nations spend more than 90% of their time indoors, that indoor concentrations of pollutants (including toxic chemicals) are often "substantially" higher than found outdoors, and that small children, the elderly, and the infirm are likely to spend all their time indoors, leading to a permanent chronic exposure to low-grade toxic factors.

In most cases, problems with a building's engineering, construction, and ventilation system are the causes. Studies suggest that symptoms occur 50% more frequently in buildings with mechanical ventilation systems. Among 2,000 office workers in Germany with work-related symptoms, there was a 50% higher than average rate of upper respiratory tract infections that were directly traceable to problems with mechanically ventilated buildings, reports Dr. Hodgson. A U.S. study found that 20% of office workers had job-related SBS symptoms, including a subjective sense of being less productive in their work.

Besides ventilation problems, other sources of indoor toxic pollution include volatile organic compounds released from particleboard desks, furniture, carpets, glues, paints, office machine toners, and perfumes. All contribute to "a complex mixture of very low levels of individual pollutants," states Dr. Hodgson. Bioaerosols are also indoor contaminants and originate as biological agents from mold spores, allergy-producing microbes, mites, or animal danders; then they are distributed through an indoor space by ventilation, heating, or air conditioning systems.

Of buildings classified as sources of SBS, one study showed that 70% have inadequate flow of fresh outside air. It also found that 50% to 70% of such buildings have poor distribution of air within the occupied space; 60% have poor filtration of outdoor pollutants; 60% have standing water that fosters biological growths; and 20% have malfunctioning humidifiers.[11]

For more on **environmental illness**, see *Alternative Medicine Guide to Chronic Fatigue, Fibromyalgia, and Environmental Illness* (Future Medicine Publishing, 1998; ISBN 1-887299-11-4); to order, call 800-333-HEAL.

For information on **the health effects of sick building syndrome**, contact: Environmental Detoxification Consultants, 413 Grassy Hill Road, Woodbury, CT 06798; tel/fax: 203-263-2970.

Treatment Options
for Environmental Illness

Many of the reactions in environmental illness involve the brain and have been treated successfully by placing either ceramic or neodymium disc magnets bitemporally. This specific type of arrangement immediately reduces most of the mental and emotional symptoms. However, as a preventive measure, also sleep on a negative magnetic field bed pad and with negative field magnets at the crown of the head.

People living near high-tension power lines can be adversely influenced by these power lines. There are two factors involved: the 60-cycle pulsing frequency, which is stressful to the body, and the sufficiently high, stressful, positive magnetic field in the immediate vicinity of these lines. For example, Kathy lived very near a transformer substation and had multiple mental and emotional symptoms. I advised her to move from this location, but for financial reasons, she could not move. However, she decided to sleep on a negative magnetic field bed pad and with four 4" x 6" x 1" ceramic magnets at her headboard. Within one week, all of her symptoms disappeared.

For the adverse health reactions from being exposed to computer screens for long periods of time, some people have reported health benefits from using "magnetic shielding." Sitting on a 4" x 6" x $\frac{1}{2}$" magnet and wearing a smaller magnet on the chest may offset the effects of EMFs.

Symptoms due to hypersensitive, chronic maladaptive reactions to chemicals are reduced or completely relieved when the symptomatic area is exposed to a negative magnetic field. Magnet therapy reduces symptoms by activating the bicarbonate buffer system, which helps maintain a normal pH. A negative magnetic field is also an energy activator of oxidoreductase enzymes, which flood the body with all the stress-relieving benefits of increased oxygen levels.

A negative magnetic field of appropriate gauss strength controls the nervous system's abnormal responses to chemicals with greater efficiency than anti-seizure medications, tranquilizers, or antidepressants, and does not produce side effects. A chemically sensitive person should sleep on a magnetic bed pad and with four 4" x 6" x 1" ceramic magnets at the headboard. Another valuable treatment is breathing negative magnetized oxygen during the night and as much as possible during the day.

Success Stories: Magnet Therapy
Helps Environmental Illness

Susan was in her fifties when she was diagnosed with environmental illness and multiple chemical sensitivity. She was referred to as a "universal reactor" because she was reactive to almost every chemical in the environment. As a treatment for this condition, she put a 2" x 2" flexible magnet over each temple (held in place with a headband, then secured with a disc magnet). Finally, she put a super neodymium magnet on the middle of her forehead, held in place with a button magnet. This negative magnetic field exposure relieved her symptoms (poor balance and brain swelling) within 30 minutes.

John, a chemically sensitive 52-year-old man, began preventive magnetic therapy in 1986. He slept on a magnetic bed pad and with four 4" x 6" x 1" ceramic magnets at the headboard. Since then, he has been able to tolerate perfumes much more than before his preventive therapy. Without magnets, some of the toxic chemicals in many perfumes destroyed his ability to think clearly. When an acute reaction occurs, he wears two ceramic disc magnets bitemporally; this arrangement keeps his brain sharp and clear for long periods.

Sarah had experienced sinus pressure, headaches, and eye focusing problems whenever she was exposed to car and diesel truck exhaust. She found a way of using magnet therapy to combat these symptoms. First, she clipped a button magnet over her hair, then fastened a super neodymium magnet against her scalp over the painful area. While driving, she discovered that wearing these magnets always served to alleviate her symptoms.

Eye Disorders

NEARLY 60% OF ALL Americans require vision correction by the time they reach adulthood, but standard treatments such as corrective lenses or surgery may in fact contribute to further visual impairment. Fortunately, many vision problems can be prevented or treated through the use of alternative therapies. Many people grow accustomed to their vision problems, assuming that their eyes are deteriorating as a result of aging. However, poor diet and nutrition, physical, mental, and emotional stress, poor visual skills, and side effects of pharmaceutical drugs are the causes of many vision problems, which are often unrelated to eye disease or to error in the functioning of the visual system.

"The proper functioning of our visual system has far-reaching effects on our general health, beyond an ability to see clearly," says Glen Swartwout, O.D., of Hilo, Hawaii. "Information processed by the eyes helps to regulate functions such as biological rhythms, as well as the nervous, endocrine, and immune systems. It also provides the dominant source

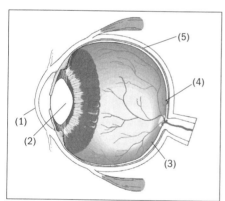

PARTS OF THE EYE. Light rays enter the eye through the cornea (1) to the lens (2) where light is focused as it travels to the retina (3). The retina, an extension of the brain, collects light through photo- or light-sensitive cells. The area of the retina with the highest concentration of photo-sensitive cells is the macula (4), responsible for central vision. Surrounding the retina is the choroid (5), which is filled with capillaries transporting nutrients to the eye.

of information for human perception, thinking, and coordination of movement."

The ability to process visual information depends upon a highly refined eye/brain communication. As light strikes the retina (the innermost layer of the eye, which receives images), chemical changes convert the light energy to a visual impulse, which is then processed by the brain. According to Dr. Swartwout, when eye/brain communication is disrupted, related problems include blurred vision, altered depth perception, loss of central or peripheral vision, double vision, sensitivity to light, and changes in color perception. If not treated, impaired vision can lead to any number of physiological or psychological problems, including lack of coordination, spatial disorientation, or reading, writing, and learning difficulties.

Dr. Swartwout notes that a great many factors can contribute to visual problems, including nutritional deficiency, alcohol, drugs, physical strain, dental problems, poor posture, environmental pollution, harmful lighting, and emotional stress. If these problems go untreated, vision disorders and eye disease can occur. He adds that "drugs and surgery do not correct or eliminate the causes of disease, which are often individual and multifactorial."

Cataracts

Defined as a partial or complete clouding of the clear lens of the eye, cataracts are the leading cause of impaired vision and blindness in the United States.[1] Though one can develop cataracts at any age, it occurs most frequently in the older adult. Dr. Swartwout notes that in addition to the aging process, risk factors include extensive exposure to radiation or infrared light, certain medications such as steroids, various injuries, and diseases. He adds that cataracts have also been linked to vitamin, mineral, and protein imbalances, and may be caused by free radicals in the eyes. Free radicals produce acids, and an acid state contributes to the production of toxins and blocks sufficient levels of oxygen in the eyes. If left untreated, this condition will severely damage the eye over a period of time.

The negative magnetic field can reverse the process. A negative magnetic field is a free-radical scavenger. That is, a negative magnetic field will quickly turn an acid state into a normal alkaline state and convert free radicals into oxygen. Moreover, a negative magnetic field also stimulates the retina of the eye to produce the hormone melatonin, a strong free-radical scavenger. As such, the negative magnetic field has been used successfully to treat cataracts in both animals and humans.

For example, Mary developed cataracts in both eyes. Her eyesight became so poor that she could not even thread a needle for her sewing projects that she loved to do daily. After her eyes were magnetically treated for several weeks, her eyesight began to improve, and she had no difficulty threading a needle.

It is important to magnetically treat the eyes whenever there is any question of cataracts, glaucoma, or macular degeneration. A good treatment for cataracts or macular degeneration is to use the magnetic eye unit, composed of a magnetic light shield with a 1" x 1/8" neodymium disc over each eye.

When treating cataracts, Dr. Swartwout stresses the relationship between nutrition and vision. For prevention, he recommends a diet consisting of unrefined, natural foods, in addition to vitamin and nutritional supplements. Conversely, refined, processed, and junk foods may contribute to the development of cataracts and glaucoma, along with stress, alcohol, caffeine, sugar, and smoking—all of which deplete the essential nutrients.

Macular Degeneration

Macular degeneration is a condition in which the macula, the central area of the retina, deteriorates, resulting in the loss of sharp vision. It is the leading cause of severe visual loss in both the U.S. and Europe for those 55 years or older, and is the third leading cause of impaired vision among those over 65.[2] In addition to aging, risk factors include atherosclerosis and hypertension. Macular degeneration may also be linked to nutritional deficiencies.

Melatonin levels are raised when treating the eyes with a magnet, because the retina produces additional melatonin in response to a negative magnetic field. Melatonin is an antioxidant hormone. At the same time, magnetically treat the body systemically to stimulate the pineal gland and intestinal tract to increase melatonin production. This is accomplished by lying on a magnetic pad at night and with four 4" x 6" x 1" ceramic magnets at the crown of the head.

For local eye treatment, use a magnetic eye unit, composed of a magnetic light shield with a 1" x 1/8" neodymium disc magnet placed on the shield over each eye. This protocol can be used as routine treatment for any eye condition.

Diabetes is a major cause of eye degeneration, encouraging the development of macular degeneration, cataracts, glaucoma, and vascular disorders of the retina. Treatment options for diabetes should be considered when treating eye disorders.

For more about **magnet therapy for diabetes**, see Diabetes.

John was a doctor who developed macular degeneration in his late sixties. He complained of having a large black spot in his vision. He improved his nutrition and began breathing magnetized oxygen from an oxygen concentrator on a regular basis. He also obtained a multi-magnet flexible mat, which he wore over his eyes at night, and slept with four 4" x 6" x 1" ceramic magnets at the crown of his head. This combined magnetic and oxygen treatment reversed his macular degeneration.

Like cataracts, macular degeneration can also be linked to nutritional deficiencies, especially among older individuals. Jonathan Wright, M.D., of Kent, Washington, and Alan Gaby, M.D., of Baltimore, Maryland, point out that there is a large body of clinical evidence suggesting that nutrient supplementation, particularly with antioxidants, may retard the aging process. According to Drs. Gaby and Wright, "With advancing age, nutritional status tends to decline because of reduced gastrointestinal absorption and impaired cellular uptake of nutrients. The sensory organs involved in vision, hearing, smell, and taste appear to be especially vulnerable to the effects of nutritional deficiency, and the purposes of supplementation are to delay the inevitable process of cellular degeneration and to enhance the function of those cells which are living."[3]

Drs. Gaby and Wright recently reviewed the role of nutritional factors in cataracts and macular degeneration, and found the following nutrients to be beneficial:[4]

■ Zinc: Necessary for normal visual function and adaptation to the dark. Zinc deficiency may lead to cataracts, and supplementation reduces visual loss in macular degeneration.

■ Selenium: Is an antioxidant, and may help prevent cataracts. Visual acuity improved in patients with macular degeneration when supplemented with selenium and vitamin E.

■ Taurine: May protect cells from harmful effects of ultraviolet light.

■ Vitamin C (ascorbic acid): One of the most important antioxidants in the eye. Supplementation can improve vision in those with cataracts.

■ Vitamin E: A deficiency of this important antioxidant may lead to cataracts. Vitamin E in large doses can prevent macular degeneration.

■ Vitamin A: Necessary for maintenance of healthy rods and cones (the visual cells of the eye) in the retina.

■ Riboflavin: Necessary co-factor for the antioxidant enzyme glutathione reductase. Riboflavin deficiency in animals leads to cataracts.

■ N-acetyl-cysteine: Has antioxidant activity and may prevent cataracts and other degenerative changes in the eye.

■ Flavonoids: A group of compounds found in plants (in particularly high concentrations in blueberries and grapes). Flavonoids have antioxidant and anti-inflammatory effects. They can help to improve night vision and adaptation to the dark, visual acuity, and capillary integrity (reduces hemorrhage in diabetic retinopathy).

Gastrointestinal Problems

PROPER DIGESTION is a requirement for optimum health. Disorders of the gastrointestinal tract are quite common and can lead to improper digestion, malabsorption, and nutritional deficiencies, all of which may contribute to the development of many other diseases. The gastrointestinal tract is a tube 25-32 feet long that begins at the mouth and ends at the anus. It comprises the mouth, pharynx, esophagus, stomach, small intestine (duodenum, jejunum, and ileum), large intestine (cecum, ascending colon, transverse colon, and descending colon), rectum, and anus. Accessory organs—the liver, pancreas, and gallbladder—all play an important role in digestion.

Digestion begins when food mixes with enzymes in saliva. The process is then carried on in the stomach by hydrochloric acid (HCl) and pepsin. Food is liquified in the stomach and passes into the small intestine, where it is further broken down by digestive enzymes from the pancreas (the enzyme protease digests proteins, amylase digests carbohydrates, and lipase digests fats). The gallbladder secretes bile, formed by the liver, to aid absorption of fats and fat-soluble vitamins. Most food absorption takes place in the small intestine, while water, electrolytes (essential body chemicals), and some of the final products of digestion are absorbed in the large intestine.

Colitis

Colitis involves inflammation of the colon. Symptoms include diarrhea, fever, weight loss, abdominal tenderness, and blood in the stool. Ulcerative colitis is characterized by open sores or lesions in the lining of the colon.

A Primer on Digestion

Digestion begins in the mouth with digestive enzymes secreted by the salivary glands. These enzymes include amylase, lipase, and some protease. Also at work in the mouth are the enzymes (plant enzymes) present in foods being eaten.

Salivary enzymes combined with the plant enzymes continue digestion in the upper (cardiac) portion of the stomach. Amylase will digest up to 60% of carbohydrates, protease up to 30% of protein, and lipase up to 10% of fat, before HCl (hydrochloric or stomach acid) and pepsin (a stomach enzyme) begin to work in the stomach.

Stomach cells secrete enough HCl to further acidify the predigested food to a low pH. This acidic pH temporarily deactivates the plant enzymes, and the predigested food passes to the lower portion of the stomach, from which cells in the stomach lining secrete more pepsin; it is here that pepsin continues the digestion of protein. Adequate HCl is required to activate pepsin from its inactive enzyme form and to maintain the stomach pH below 3.0, the optimum level for pepsin to work.

In the next stage of digestion, the partially digested food and deactivated plant enzymes pass into the upper part of the small intestine (the duodenum). Here, digestion continues with the help of bile, pancreatic enzymes, and an alkalizing substance (bicarbonate) that

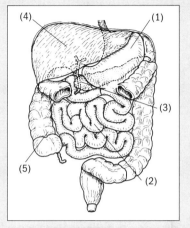

THE DIGESTIVE SYSTEM. Digestion begins in the mouth, then food travels to the stomach (1), where it is further broken down by gastric juices. Next, the partially digested food goes to the small intestine (2) where enzymes from the pancreas (3) and bile produced by the liver (4) act upon the food to extract nutrients for absorption into blood and lymph cells. The unusable food materials are sent to the large intestine (5) for evacuation from the body.

reactivates the food enzymes by reducing acidity. Then digestion proceeds to the jejunum (the next section of the small intestine), where disaccharidases (sugar-digesting enzymes) are secreted. From the small intestine, the majority of nutrients from digested food are absorbed into the blood.

Bleeding ulcerative colitis can be successfully treated with a negative magnetic field. Use the 11" x 17" multi-purpose magnetic pad, worn day or night. Place a 4" x 6" x ¹/₂" ceramic magnet on top of the pad, directly over the lesion, to increase depth of penetration. Hold in place with a 4" x 52" body wrap.

It is important to understand that when the intestinal tract is in a negative magnetic field, the involuntary muscle movement necessary for proper passage of food through the tract is slowed down. So, when magnetically treating the stomach and intestines, the negative magnetic field has to be removed for one hour after each meal. In addition, since colitis and many other intestinal syndromes directly relate to maladaptive reactions to foods, it is important to rotate all foods on a four-day diversified basis.

John, 65, had chronic colitis produced by a viral infection. He was literally starving and dehydrated from frequent diarrhea. The illness was so advanced that he required intravenous feeding. A plastiform magnet strip was placed on his abdomen. The magnet stopped the peristalsis and thus the diarrhea. However, the magnet had to be periodically removed in order for John to have a regular bowel movement. Gradually, the magnet was removed for brief periods of time, until finally he could go several hours without diarrhea. His condition improved significantly and remained well controlled with the application of magnetic therapy for one hour, three times a day.

For the **Four-Day Diversified Rotation Diet**, see Appendix.

Since many gastrointestinal disorders share symptoms such as inflammation, poor absorption, bloating, gas, abdominal cramps, constipation, and diarrhea, the treatments often overlap. The alternative approach to such disorders includes dietary restrictions, nutritional supplementation, detection and elimination of maladaptive reactions to food and stress reduction.

Constipation

Defined as infrequent or difficult evacuation of fecal material (stools), constipation is most often caused by lack of fiber and fluids in the diet. A low intestinal population of the beneficial bacteria *acidophilus*, magnesium deficiency, iron supplementation, and taking painkillers or antidepressants can also produce constipation. It is important to have at least one bowel movement per day. This avoids the formation and absorption of toxic by-products produced by poor digestion and assimilation.

The 5" x 12" double magnet, multi-magnet flexible mat, placed crosswise on the body, is suitable for treating constipation. On top of this mat, place a 4" x 6" x ½" magnet lengthwise. An alternative is to use the 4" x 12" plastiform magnet with a 4" x 6" x ½" magnet on the

Treating Food Maladaptive Reactions

It is always preferable to prevent any food maladaptive reaction. In order to accomplish this, one must understand that a repetitive diet of a few frequently eaten foods most often causes the development of maladaptive reactions. Researchers have found that the diets of allergy patients normally consist of less than 30 foods that are eaten repeatedly. These 30 foods then become the basis for the most common food intolerances. The likelihood of having a maladaptive reaction to any given food is often directly proportional to how often the person eats that food. One can alleviate the problems associated with such a monotonous and repetitive diet by following a Four-Day Diversified Rotation Diet.

All addictive (immunologic and non-immunologic) reactions produce acidity in the body. Because exposure to a negative magnetic field alkalinizes the body, magnets should be used to treat the acidity produced by food addictions. The local area of symptoms should first be treated with a negative field magnet that is slightly larger than the area. At the same time, the brain should be treated with a negative field (bitemporal placement of either the ceramic or neodymium disc magnets). Treatment usually requires a minimum of ten minutes, but it may take hours or even days to heal the damage from these reactions.

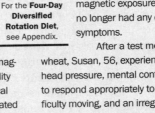

For the **Four-Day Diversified Rotation Diet**, see Appendix.

After eating a test meal of blackberries, Bruce, 14, complained of stomach upset, headache, and irritability. He was treated immediately with a negative magnetic field. Specifically, he used 4" x 12" plastiform strips, one on the abdomen and another down the spine, as well as 1½" x ¼" ceramic disc magnets on both temples. After 30 minutes, he relaxed to the point of sleep, and his headache and irritability were entirely alleviated.

Tom, 7, complained of headache, stomach upset, and pain behind his knees after a test meal of wheat. He was treated with a bitemporal placement of ceramic magnets, as well as plastiform magnetic strips on the abdomen, back, and behind the knees. Thirty minutes after this magnetic exposure, Tom said he no longer had any of his original symptoms.

After a test meal of buckwheat, Susan, 56, experienced a vise-like head pressure, mental confusion, inability to respond appropriately to questions, difficulty moving, and an irregular pulse. The negative field side of a 4" x 6" x ½" ceramic magnet was placed under the back of her head for approximately 30 minutes. Five minutes later, her eyes were open and she felt mentally clear. She was able to sit up and alert enough to talk. Even after the magnet was removed, her symptoms did not return and her pulse normalized.

center. This arrangement should held in place with a 4" x 52" body wrap. The negative magnetic field will ultimately pull fecal matter and fluid down into the rectal area. Subsequently, the person will have an urge for a bowel movement immediately upon awakening in the morning.

General Magnet Placement for Gastrointestinal Problems

■ Epigastric Placement—There are two reasons for treating the epigastric area (upper middle region of the abdomen): to help handle withdrawal symptoms caused by maladaptive reactions to specific foods and to heal a hiatal hernia or gastric ulcer. Since gastric ulcers frequently relate to infections in the stomach, it is ideal to treat 24 hours per day, because the longer the exposure, the more significant the therapeutic value. However, remove the magnets from the epigastric area after meals and keep them off for one hour to allow for peristalsis. When lying down, use the 4" x 6" x ½" ceramic block magnet. Otherwise, use either a 5" x 6" or 5" x 12" double magnet, multi-magnet flexible mat (held in place with a 4" x 52" body wrap). Even better, place a 4" x 6" x ½" ceramic magnet on top of the mat.

■ Large Intestine Placement—The large intestine can be treated with 5" x 12" double magnet, multi-magnet flexible mats. The 11" x 17" multipurpose pad composed of mini-block magnets is also useful for treating the abdomen. Whenever lying down, a 4" x 6" x ½" ceramic magnet can be worn on top of this mat, directly over the affected area. This arrangement is suitable for treating Crohn's disease, intestinal parasites, and fungal infections.

■ Rectal-Genital Placement—The rectal-genital placement of magnets is useful for treating hemorrhoids or infections in the lower colon. Whenever sitting down, place a 4" x 6" x ½" magnet lengthwise along the body under the rectal-genital area. This exposure should be maintained daily for as many hours as possible and can be combined with a pelvic placement of the same type of magnet for added benefits. The comfort chair pad with mini-block magnets in the seat and back cushion also has a substantial therapeutic value.

Nutritional considerations related to constipation include the amount of liquid and fiber in the diet as well as how much vitamin C is being taken. When treating constipation, drink 10-12 glasses of fluid a day and immediately increase the amount of fiber in the diet. Vitamin C can also be taken in amounts up to bowel tolerance. A vitamin C flush is better than an enema or colonic—take one tablespoon of vitamin C each hour until an intestinal flush occurs.

Diverticulitis

Diverticulosis is a condition in which the walls of the intestines balloon out forming pouches. A small percentage of these patients go on to develop diverticulitis, an inflammation of these pouches. Problems occur when undigested food particles lodge in these pouches. This causes irritation and can lead to inflammation.

Diverticulitis should be treated vigorously with a negative magnetic field. Use a 5" x 12" double magnet, multi-magnet flexible mat with one or two 4" x 6" x ½" magnets on top. An 11" x 17" multi-purpose pad is also useful for treating the abdomen. This magnetic arrangement needs to stay in place most of the time, except for an hour or so, two or three times a day, when it is removed for the sake of digestion and bowel movements.

Parasites

A parasite is any organism that lives off another organism (called a host) and draws nourishment from it. Specifically, parasites are the protozoa (single-cell organisms), arthropods (insects), and worms that infect the body and cause serious damage to tissues and organs. Common forms of the protozoan parasites are *Giardia lamblia*, which causes giardiasis; *Entamoeba histolytica*, which causes dysentery; and *Cryptosporidium*, which causes diarrhea, particularly in people with immunologic diseases such as AIDS. The most common arthropod parasites are lice, mites, ticks, and fleas. Worm parasites include pinworms, roundworms, tapeworms, whipworms, hookworms, and filaria (threadlike worms that inhabit the blood and tissues).

Parasites are inhibited by a negative magnetic field. Since some parasites in the colon are anaerobic (grow in the absence of molecular oxygen), an increased oxygen supply—created by magnetic exposure—inhibits their replication. In order to eliminate parasites, treat the abdomen with a 11" x 17" multipurpose magnet pad. Place a 4" x 6" x ½" magnet on top of the mat. The magnets should be worn as much as possible, but they must be removed for one hour after meals.

Hiatal Hernia

In this condition, a portion of the cardia (the upper part of the stomach) bulges through the gap in the diaphragm into the esophagus. Symptoms include esophageal reflux, epigastric pain, regurgitation, and severe burning (heartburn) that is worse when lying down. This can eventually lead to an ulcer. Routinely go on a Four-Day Diversified Rotation Diet. Symptomatic relief can be achieved by placing a 4" x 6" x ½" magnet directly over the epigastric area.

For the **Four-Day Diversified Rotation Diet**, see Appendix.

Indigestion and Nausea

Pains in the stomach, nausea, vomiting, or abdominal pains are usually caused by maladaptive reactions to foods. The first treatment option is the Four-Day Diversified Rotation

Diet. Also, place a 4" x 6" x ½" magnet over the area of discomfort in the abdominal area. Usually, this type of treatment reverses the symptoms within ten to 30 minutes.

Magnetic therapy has been used to relieve stomach cramps and nausea in many patients. Jan was helped considerably when she had severe bouts of gastritis. While lying on her back, she applied the negative field side of a 4" x 6" x ½" ceramic magnet over her stomach. This created a gurgling sensation and a feeling of normal flow within her digestive system. She then moved the magnets lower, which accelerated the healing process and helped her to expel gas. Upon doing so, the stomach pain was eliminated.

Susan, 57, had an extreme case of nausea. She found that her symptoms were eliminated when she placed a 4" x 6" x ½" ceramic magnet over her stomach. This negative magnetic field exposure eliminated all her symptoms within 20 minutes.

Irritable Bowel Syndrome

Irritable bowel syndrome (IBS) is a condition in which the large intestine, or colon, fails to operate normally. It is a functional disorder, since there is no evidence of structural damage to the intestine. Symptoms include pain, constipation, diarrhea, gas, nausea, anorexia, and anxiety or depression.[1] Of the patients I've tested, all cases of IBS have been due to maladaptive food reactions. Treatment of IBS aims to reduce the irritation to the digestive system and therefore relies on dietary changes.

For maladaptive reactions to foods, the abdomen should be treated with a suitable size negative magnetic field. Use the 11" x 17" multi-purpose pad; usually a 4" x 6" x ½" ceramic magnet needs to be placed on top of the other magnets. The magnets can be worn as much as needed, but they need to be removed for one hour after meals. It is imperative to rotate the foods on a Four-Day Diversified Rotation Diet.

Heart Disease

THE UNITED STATES leads the world in death rates from heart disease. Heart disease has been the leading killer of Americans nearly every year since 1900, now causing half of all U.S. deaths.[1] Among the conditions included are coronary heart disease (decreased blood flow to the heart usually caused by atherosclerosis), congestive heart failure (cardiomyopathy), heart attack (myocardial infarction), chest pain (angina pectoris), high blood pressure (hypertension), arrhythmia, rheumatic heart disease, and hardening of the arteries (arteriosclerosis, of which atherosclerosis, involving fatty arterial wall deposits, is the most common).

According to the American Heart Association (AHA), every 33 seconds an American dies of cardiovascular disease (CVD)—that's about 954,000 deaths annually or about 42% of all mortalities. Every 20 seconds, an American suffers a heart attack, and every 60 seconds, somebody dies from one, reports AHA. Among deaths attributed to CVD, 52.3% are women and 47.7% are men. African Americans suffer CVD at much higher rates than whites: the rate of death from CVD among black males is 47.4% higher and among black females, it's 69.1% higher.

A common precursor of heart disease is atherosclerosis, or thickening of the arterial walls. In atherosclerosis, the inner arterial walls harden and thicken due to deposits of fatty substances. These substances form a plaque that, with buildup, causes a narrowing of the arteries.[2] Over time, plaque can block the arteries and interrupt blood flow to the organs they supply, including the heart and brain. Atherosclerosis of the coronary arteries (the arteries supplying the muscle of the heart), known as coronary heart disease, is one of the most common forms of heart disease in the U.S. today. Coronary heart disease can lead to heart attack, coronary

Types of Heart Disease

Angina Pectoris—Characterized by discomfort, heaviness, pain, or pressure in the chest, angina results from a diminished supply of oxygen to the heart muscle. Angina is a warning sign of heart attack risk.

Atherosclerosis—The most common form of artheriosclerosis (hardening of the arterial walls), atherosclerosis involves deposits of fatty substances on the walls of the arteries causing them to thicken. In advanced stages, blood flow is impeded. In peripheral arteriosclerosis, the extremities, especially the legs, are frequently involved, and the aorta is often the site of a general thickening of the arterial wall. Plaques tend to form on the arterial wall where arteries branch from the aorta. When these atheromatous plaques form, specific organs or extremities may have a reduced blood supply.

Heart Attack—A heart attack (myocardial infarction) occurs when blood supply and the oxygen it carries to the heart is cut off to the point that part of the heart literally dies. If blockage is extensive, death can result.

Congestive Heart Failure—Medically termed cardiomyopathy, this condition literally means failure of the heart muscle. When the heart has been weakened by a heart attack, for example, it is unable to pump fully, resulting in blood congestion in the heart. A typical sign of congestive heart failure is shortness of breath either with minimal exertion or when lying down at night.

High Blood Pressure—High blood pressure or hypertension is the most common cardiovascular disease in industrialized nations. It weakens and degenerates arteries and is a major cause of heart attack, stroke, and congestive heart failure. In the large number of hypertensive patients I've examined, the central cause has been maladaptive reactions to frequently eaten food, usually due to food addictions.

occlusion, and angina while atherosclerosis of the cerebral arteries (the arteries that supply blood to the brain) can precipitate strokes. Coronary occlusion and heart attacks can, in turn, lead to another heart condition, congestive heart failure.

Success Story: Magnet Therapy for Atherosclerosis

Magnetic therapy demonstrated excellent results in a case of atherosclerosis resulting from diabetes. John, 70, with atherosclerotic heart disease, underwent a multiple bypass operation. Two years later, his heart pain returned, leaving him unsteady on his feet and subject to disorientation in familiar surroundings. His speech grew thick and he became chronically depressed. He slept with the negative field of several ceramic magnets placed at the crown of his head. John also continually wore a magnet strapped to his skin over his heart during the day. Within a week, his symptoms improved and, after one month of this treatment, he had no heart pain. Plus, his balance returned, his speech became distinct once again, his depression disappeared completely, and his mental confusion was remarkably reduced.

Success Story: Magnets Help Avoid Surgery

Betty, 83, had a major coronary artery that was 80% blocked. For two months prior to her scheduled operation (angioplasty) for the artery, Betty slept on a magnetic bed and wore a magnet over her heart during the day. When the time arrived for the operation, the blockage was so markedly reduced that the procedure was cancelled.

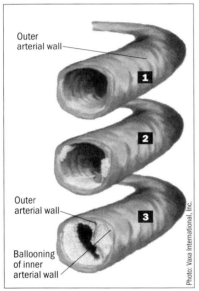

Outer arterial wall

Outer arterial wall

Ballooning of inner arterial wall

Photo: Vaxa International, Inc.

How Arteries Thicken
1. A normal, healthy artery with open and clear passages.
2. The beginning of cholesterol plaque buildup within the artery. The inner artery wall is also beginning to weaken and bulge with cholesterol and toxic deposits.
3. Severely restricted artery with cholesterol plaque filling the majority of the passage. Note further breakdown and ballooning of inner artery wall.

What Causes Heart Disease?

Maladaptive food reactions, especially food addiction, are the main culprits in heart disease. The standard American diet (refined, processed foods, saturated fats, and high levels of red meat and dairy products) and lifestyle are other factors.

There is a significant body of evidence that homocysteine, a normal by-product of protein metabolism, may play a role in artherosclerosis (hardening of the arteries). Homocysteine is normally converted into a harmless amino acid (cystathionine). But in some individuals, a genetic defect or nutritional deficiency (in folic acid and the B vitamins) prevents the normal conversion process of homocysteine from occurring. Excess homocysteine may generate free radicals, which are capable of oxidizing cholesterol and damaging arterial walls.

There are two kinds of cholesterol: low-density lipoprotein or LDL, and high-density lipoprotein

or HDL (SEE QUICK DEFINITION). LDL cholesterol becomes harmful only after it has been oxidized by free radicals from high levels of homocysteine, dietary sources (such as processed foods
high in trans-fatty acids), or exposure to environmental chemicals. Oxidized LDL initiates the
formation of plaque on arterial walls, interfering
with blood circulation and leading to artherosclerosis and ultimately to heart attacks and strokes.[3]

While medical research has been focusing on
multiple predisposing factors for atherosclerosis
and arteriosclerosis, there is a central factor that
has been largely ignored—acidity. The amino
acids and calcium that form plaques are soluble in
an alkaline medium, but become insoluble in high
acidity. The acidity is caused by maladaptive reactions, mostly to foods but to a lesser degree with
chemicals. A negative magnetic field can help
resolve the insoluble amino acids and calcium.

Treatment Options for Heart Disease

A negative magnetic field oxygenates and alkalinizes body tissues and cells. These two actions
oppose the acidity required for the creation of
insoluble amino acid and calcium deposits in
existing plaques. Since a negative magnetic field
has a local effect, magnets must be applied directly over the plaques in order to achieve therapeutic results.

Experience has convinced me that magnetic
treatment for arterial disease is more reliable and
beneficial than EDTA chelation. However, magnetic treatment needs to be continuous in order
to resolve arteriosclerosis and may take weeks or
even months. I have repeatedly observed immediate relief of any pain associated with vascular
spasms or blocked arteries. This pain is most
often caused by a reduction of oxygen to tissues, so a negative magnetic

QUICK DEFINITION

Lipoproteins occur in two principal forms: low- and high-density. Low-density lipoproteins (LDLs), which are made from protein and fat molecules, circulate in the blood and act as the primary carriers of cholesterol to the cells of the body. An elevated level of LDL, often called "bad" cholesterol, contributes to atherosclerosis, a circulatory system disease that leads to a buildup of plaque deposits on the inner walls of the arteries. These plaque deposits can eventually cause heart attacks, stroke, and other illnesses. A diet high in saturated fats can increase levels of LDLs in the blood. High-density lipoproteins (HDLs) contain a larger amount of protein and less fat than LDLs. HDLs readily absorb cholesterol and related compounds in the blood and transport them to the liver for elimination. HDL, or "good" cholesterol, may also be able to take cholesterol from plaque deposits on the artery walls, thus helping to reverse the process of atherosclerosis. A higher ratio of HDL to LDL cholesterol in the blood is associated with a reduced risk of cardiovascular disease.

A **trans-fatty acid (TFA)** is a chemically and structurally altered hydrogenated vegetable oil (such as margarine), which is combined with hydrogen to lengthen shelf-life. Commercially prepared hydrogenated fats are from 8% to 70% trans-fatty acids which comprise about 60% of the fat found in processed foods. TFAs can increase the risk of heart disease by 27% when consumed as at least 12% of the total fat intake. TFAs also reduce production of prostaglandins (hormones that act locally to control all cell-to-cell interactions) and interfere with fatty acid metabolism.

field reverses this deficiency of oxygen and prevents tissue damage.

Treatment must emphasize the reversal of food addictions and allergies, as well as optimal nutritional support, as a starting point. For someone with cardiovascular disease, any diet program should include not only the Four-Day Rotation Diet but also a high-fiber, low-fat diet, and very low in artificial chemicals. Seek the professional advice of a nutritionally oriented physician in order to reverse all potential nutrient deficiencies.

Begin magnet therapy by sleeping with magnets at the crown of the head, using four 4" x 6" x 1" magnets placed $^3/_4$" apart in a row, so that the head is in the magnetic field during sleep. In addition, sleep on a negative magnetic field bed pad (mini-block magnets that are $1^7/_8$" x $^7/_8$" x $^3/_4$" placed two inches apart).

For optimum therapeutic results, the magnet needs to be large enough and of sufficient gauss strength to penetrate the affected area. The stronger the magnetic field, the better are the results. Ceramic magnets are capable of penetrating into the body's organs such as the heart. The double magnet, multi-magnet flexible mat (composed of strips of plastiform magnets) is ideal for lesions within two inches of the surface. Use this as a foundation for the ceramic magnets.

While local treatment is beneficial, there is mounting evidence that systemic treatment of the body is also helpful. Joan, for example, developed a blood clot in the left groin after the birth of her child, and had to wear an elastic stocking that kept this leg under pressure. In spite of this, a tender area in the left groin the size of a marble developed. For 35 years, she had difficulty when walking upstairs, only able to take a couple of steps before her leg would start hurting due to the reduced blood supply. Joan decided to try a 12-month test of sleeping on a magnetic bed pad. She also slept with magnets in a carrier at the crown of her head. After twelve months, she could walk up a flight of stairs without any pain. A physical examination showed that the painful, enlarged area in the left groin was no longer present.

The Four-Day Diversified Rotation Diet is necessary to reverse any degenerative disease, including heart diseases of all kinds. The reason is because any maladaptive reaction to foods or chemicals produces inflammation, acidity, and a deficiency of oxygen. Then, target tissues like the arteries develop problems associated with all the vascular diseases. Stress, infections, and nutritional deficiencies further compromise the body. This entire metabolic process, including acidity, inflammation, infection, and low tissue oxygen, can be reduced by combining magnetic therapy with a Four-Day Diversified Rotation Diet and nutritional supplementation.

For the **Four-Day Diversified Rotation Diet**, see Appendix.

Nutritional Supplements for Heart Disease

Possibly the most important nutritional fact to understand regarding the heart is the role of magnesium. All muscles in the body require this mineral for their ability to rest after contraction, but as the heart is a muscle that never stops working, it requires an estimated eight times the amount of magnesium needed by other muscles in the body.

A healthy diet emphasizing whole, unprocessed foods (including fruits, vegetables, and sources of essential fatty acids) can reduce the risk of developing heart disease. Specifically, essential fatty acids have demonstrated the ability to reduce hypertension.[4]

Nutritional formulas designed for the cardiovascular system are an easy method of providing your heart with supplemental support for optimal functioning. A good formula will include most or all of the following: antioxidants such as coenzyme Q10; vitamins A, C, E, and B complex (B6, B12, and folic acid), selenium, and quercetin; the minerals magnesium, potassium, and calcium; and bromelain (enzymes derived from pineapple). Sufficient levels of B vitamins will prevent accumulation of toxic levels of homocysteine, while antioxidants will neutralize free radicals and prevent damage to the heart's arterial wall.

Coenzyme Q10 and vitamin E are particularly beneficial supplements for cardiovascular and coronary heart diseases, as evidenced by a large body of research. CoQ10 helps increase exercise capacity, reduce arrhythmias (irregular heartbeat), improve oxygen delivery to the heart, and enhance healing and recovery in patients with heart and circulatory problems.[5] Vitamin E provides antioxidant protection, reduces platelet aggregation or stickiness (a factor in atherosclerosis), and lowers cholesterol, all of which contribute to the prevention of cardiovascular disease.[6]

Specific Area Treatment

Cerebral Arteriosclerosis—Place a 5" x 6" double magnet, multi-magnet mat over the front of the neck. In addition, place a ceramic disc over each carotid artery (on each side of the trachea). Hold these in place with a 2" x 26" self-fastening band.

Treat the upper back of the neck and low occiput (back of the skull) with a 4" x 6" x $\frac{1}{2}$" ceramic magnet. This arrangement will treat arteries at the base of the brain, and it should take place part of the time while asleep.

Treat the temporal area, forehead, and eyes at night with the 4" x 6" x $\frac{1}{2}$" ceramic magnet. In addition, treat the spine with a 5" x 12" double magnet, multi-magnet flexible mat on the lumbar, thoracic, or cervical areas as indicated by symptoms of pain or tension. The Sleep Enhancer system (four 4" x 6" x 1" ceramic magnets, placed $\frac{3}{4}$" apart in a wooden carrier) should be used during sleep; the top of the head should be as close as possible to these magnets.

Cardiac Pain and Irregularity—During the day, place a 5" x 6" double magnet, multi-magnet flexible magnetic mat over the heart. For pain relief, place a 4" x 6" x $\frac{1}{2}$" ceramic magnet over the mat for a few minutes. It is important to emphasize that the acute phase of cardiac ischemia or coronary occlusion is a medical emergency that requires careful medical intervention beyond the use of magnetic energy. Use the 4" x 6" x $\frac{1}{2}$" ceramic magnet during the acute phase of coronary occlusion.

Heart Arrhythmia—Cardiac irregularities are often helped if maladaptive reactions to foods, chemicals, or inhalants are eliminated. If there are any maladaptive reactions, the negative magnetic field usually reduces the symptoms immediately. Chronic irregularities, on the other hand, require prolonged magnetic treatment. As a general rule, treat the heart, especially if you are over age 40, with a 5" x 6" double magnet, multi-magnet flexible mat, pinned to the clothing.

Arteriosclerosis with an Aneurysm in the Leg—An aneurysm (blood clot) is a local manifestation of the development of general arteriosclerosis. Place a 5" x 12" double magnet, flexible mat around the leg at the site of the pain, held in place with a 26" band. Another 5" x 12" flexible magnetic mat can be placed on the other side of the leg. In addition, place a 4" x 6" x $\frac{1}{2}$" magnet on this affected area. If possible, place the leg on one of the 4" x 6" x $\frac{1}{2}$" magnets when sleeping or sitting down. Place a 4" x 6" x 1" magnet on the groin area. Sleep on a magnetic bed pad and with magnets at the crown of the head. During the day, sit on a comfort chair pad composed of mini-block magnets and wear a conveniently sized multi-magnet flexible mat over the heart.

Arteriosclerotic Heart Disease—First, place a 5" x 12" double magnet, flexible mat over the heart and chest. Place on top of this six mini-block magnets ($1\frac{7}{8}$" x $\frac{7}{8}$" x $\frac{3}{8}$"), $1\frac{1}{2}$" apart crosswise in two rows. Hold in place with a 4" x 52" body wrap. An alternative to the mat is using a 4" x 6" x $\frac{1}{2}$" ceramic magnet over the heart.

Treat the brain at night by treating one side of the head with a 4" x 6" x $\frac{1}{2}$" ceramic magnet. When sitting down, sit on a comfort chair pad. Sleep on a magnetic bed pad and with magnets at the crown of the head. All patients suffering from arteriosclerosis and heart disease should use the Four-Day Diversified Rotation Diet.

For the **Four-Day Diversified Rotation Diet**, see Appendix.

Infections

INFECTIONS INVOLVE THE GROWTH of disease-causing organisms (bacteria, viruses, fungi) anywhere in the body. They can damage cells through a variety of routes, such as directly, through release of toxins, or through allergic reaction. Many of the symptoms of the infection are usually a result of the immune system mounting a response to these foreign colonies. Symptoms include redness, inflammation, pain, swelling, and formation of pus-filled pockets (abscess) at the site of the infection. If fever and painful joints occur, this may be a sign of an infectious disease that is spreading throughout the body and a health-care practitioner should be seen at once.

Conventional medical science relies on antibiotics, but they have serious side effects and are proving ineffective against newly developing resistant strains of bacteria. A negative magnetic field has a very strong and universal antibiotic effect against invading, disease-producing microorganisms. It appears that "the magnetic antibiotic" works regardless of the type or strain of bacteria, fungus, or virus. While the effectiveness of magnetic therapy in treating infections cannot be announced as scientific fact until there are more published studies, it is justifiable, based on clinical observations, to add magnetic therapy to existing therapies. In the case of minor infections that are not life-threatening, magnetic therapy should be considered the first option.

Bacteria and other infectious microorganisms replicate rapidly, and their energy life cycle is controlled primarily by a positive magnetic field. In fact, a positive magnetic field actually encourages microorganism replication.[1] On the other hand, a negative magnetic field reduces and even prevents microorganism replication.[2] This is because a well-oxygenated, highly alkalinized, and energized human biological system, all of which occurs with a negative magnetic field exposure, is capable of preventing the spread of infectious microorganisms. This was confirmed in a study from the New Jersey Institute of Technology, which involved various magnetic exposures to bacterial cultures. The response to a positive magnetic field was an increase in bacterial metabolism, while a negative magnetic field led to a decrease.[3]

The majority of microorganisms make their ATP life energy by fermentation. Fermentation, as we know, requires an acid medium and reduced amount of oxygen. In the presence of an optimum supply of oxygen and alkalinity, the microorganisms die. This is why a negative magnetic field, which maintains alkaline-hyperoxia, has an antibiotic effect on microorganisms.

A negative magnetic field is also an antibiotic for aerobic microorganisms, but in a different way. Microorganisms have a higher mineral content and higher pulsing frequency than human cells. A positive magnetic field supports this higher frquency of microorganisms, whereas a negative magnetic field supports the slower frequency of human cells. A negative magnetic field from an external static magnet helps human cells fight infections.

Success Stories: Magnets Alleviate Infections

Mary had candidiasis of the vagina and colon, which required constant antibiotic treatment. She also had frequent urinary bladder infections, again requiring antibiotics. Frustrated by her unsatisfactory results, she then exposed her pelvic area to a negative magnetic field, and both the candidiasis and urinary infections disappeared permanently.

Jim complained of a painful tooth. An examination showed pus oozing around this tooth, a clear indication of a localized infection. Placing a negative magnetic field on his face over the tooth resolved the pain in ten minutes. Furthermore, while waiting four days for his dental appointment, he kept the negative magnetic field over this tooth—when the dentist performed an examination, there was no evidence of infection.

During a flu epidemic, Susan developed characteristic flu symptoms with profuse mucous drainage from the sinuses, coughing, and general malaise. Her lungs, sinuses, and head were treated 24 hours a day with 4" x 6" x $^1/_2$" ceramic magnets. By the third day, she had no symptoms and the magnets were removed. After this, her symptoms still did not return. At the same time, a large number of people in the same community had a severe three-week siege of influenza; those patients who used magnetic therapy like Susan achieved the same results.

Treatment Options for Infections

Microorganisms, such as bacteria, fungi, and viruses, have an opposite energy system to the normal (oxidation) energy system. In fact, oxygen interferes with their enzymatic method of energy production. The body can defeat these microorganisms on the basis of this fact. Oxygen has long been noted for its suppression of infectious states, correction of disordered immunity, and production of human metabolic energy.[4] When functioning normally, our oxidative method of energy production is ten times more efficient and effective than the fermentation method used by microorganisms. A well-oxygenated human energy system is able to defeat infectious microorganisms.

The negative magnetic field's power to oxygenate as well as alkalinize bodily tissues is its key to defeating infections of all kinds. Keep in mind, however, that the magnetic field must always be negative. In addition, the magnetic field must always be larger than the infected area being treated and exposure must be as continuous as possible.

For protection against infections, sleep on a negative magnetic field bed pad, composed of $1^7/_8$" x $^7/_8$" x $^3/_8$" mini-block magnets placed $1^1/_2$" apart throughout the pad; place this pad on top of your mattress. Sleep on this pad every night, and use it continuously for any acute illness, such as influenza, colds, and pneumonia.

The crown of the head should be exposed to a negative magnetic field, using four 4" x 6" x 1" ceramic magnets placed $^3/_4$" apart in a row, and held in a carrier against the headboard. These magnets can be raised or lowered, depending on the height of the pillow. Place the head as close to the magnets as possible. While awake, use $1^1/_2$" x $^1/_2$" ceramic discs placed bitemporally. The brain responds to any abnormal response in the body, such as toxins from infections, so treating the brain is recommended.

Treating the lungs with a negative magnetic field magnetizes the oxygen concentrated in the lungs—this magnetized oxygen then circulates to the entire body. Place a 5" x 12" double magnet, multi-magnet flexible mat across the lungs on the chest and hold in place with a 4" x 52" body wrap with shoulder straps. For an acute infection in the lungs, place a 4" x 6" x $^1/_2$" magnet on top of this mat, directly over the infected area. These magnets can be held in place with the body wrap, or a specially designed garment with pockets to hold the magnets.

Heart treatment enables the cellular elements of the blood—that is, the water and oxygen flowing through the heart—to receive a negative magnetic field. In this way, the health-giving attributes of the negative magnetic field are carried throughout the entire body. Wear a 5" x 6" double magnet, multi-magnet flexible mat over the heart; this mat can be pinned to the underwear or outer clothing or held in place with a 4" x 52" body wrap.

Treating Local Infections

Local areas of fungal infections, such as candidiasis of the vagina or colon, should be treated with daily and nightly magnetic exposure with ceramic magnets. Whenever sitting down, sit on a magnetic comfort chair pad. Also, sleep at night with a 5" x 12" double magnet, multi-magnet flexible mat on the lower abdominal area. On top of this mat, place a 4" x 6" x $\frac{1}{2}$" ceramic magnet, held in place with a 4" x 52" body wrap.

If an infection is below the skin or in an organ, then a ceramic magnet that provides deep penetration must be used for treatment. A good method is to first place either a 5" x 6" or 5" x 12" double magnet, multi-magnet flexible mat over the area. Over this mat, place a ceramic magnet in one of the following sizes: $1\frac{1}{2}$" x $\frac{1}{2}$"; 2" x 5" x $\frac{1}{2}$"; 4" x 6" x $\frac{1}{2}$" (weighs 2 lbs); or 4" x 6" x 1" (weighs 4 lbs). The best way to secure the magnets is with a garment supported from the shoulders, with pockets that hold the magnets over the infection.

Bacterial and viral infections often invade the sinuses, nose, and nasal pharynx. These infections can spread to the rest of the body, so it is important to routinely treat them. When sleeping, use the magnetic eye unit and place two 1" x $\frac{1}{8}$" neodymium discs over each of the four sinuses.

During the day, tape a disc over the sinus with HY or other suitable tape; keep in place for a minimum of 14 days.

For fungal infections, such as candidiasis, or bacterial infections in the lower colon or vagina, magnets can be used to treat the pelvic area. Use a comfort chair pad, made of mini-block magnets placed $1\frac{1}{2}$" apart throughout the seat and back. The more hours of sitting on this pad, the better. When sitting down on the pad, slip a 4" x 6" x $\frac{1}{2}$" ceramic magnet under the chair seat so that it is under the genital/rectal area. At the same time, take a 4" x 6" x $\frac{1}{2}$" ceramic magnet and place it on the pelvic area. At night, place a 5" x 12" double magnet, multi-magnet flexible mat across the body on the abdominal area. On top and in the center of this mat, place a 4" x 6" x $\frac{1}{2}$" magnet lengthwise to the body, held in place with a 4" x 52" body wrap. This method is effective in treating candidiasis, bacterial infections, urinary bladder infections, parasitic infections of the colon, and genital parasitic infections.

Drinking water can be magnetized by placing a glass of water on the negative field of a 4" x 6" x $^1/_2$" ceramic magnet for at least five minutes. Drink this magnetized water to dispense a negative magnetic field throughout the body. Oxygen can also be magnetized before it is breathed, by using an oxygen concentrator. Expose the oxygen concentrator's tubing to the negative magnetic field of a 4" x 6" x 1" ceramic magnet. This procedure has a powerful effect in treating the body systemically as well as the nasal pharynx and sinuses locally. It can be used continuously in acute infectious situations, especially those of the lungs.

Additional Magnetic Treatments for Infections

■ For eye infections, use a magnetic eye unit.

■ For infected teeth or gums, place a $1^7/_8$" x $^7/_8$" x $^3/_8$" mini-block magnet on the face, directly over the infected area. It is also possible to use either a neodymium disc, which is 1" across, or a ceramic disc, which is $1^1/_2$" across. These can be either taped on the area or held in place with a 2" x 26" band.

■ For athlete's foot, place a 4" x 12" plastiform magnet, or a magnet that is at least as long as the foot, in a sock. Sleep all night with the foot against this magnet. Always use a negative magnetic field. Also, you can use negative magnetic field shoe insoles.

■ For fungal infections of the nails, magnetic treatment involves a 1" x $^1/_8$" neodymium disc, taped over the infected nail. This treatment should be done at least every night and, when convenient, also during the daytime.

■ For genital herpes, always treat with a negative magnetic field. Use the 1" x $^1/_8$" neodymium disc taped directly over the infected area. At the same time, place a 4" x 6" x $^1/_2$" magnet over the lumbar-sacral (in the pelvis, just above the tailbone) area, held in place with a 4" x 52" body wrap.

■ For throat infections, such as laryngitis, place a 5" x 6" double magnet, flexible mat around the front of the neck, held in place with a 2" x 26" self-fastening band. On top of this mat, place a ceramic disc magnet directly over the infected area.

■ For stomach infections and ulcers, place a 4" x 6" x $^1/_2$" ceramic magnet directly over the epigastric area, applied continuously for 14 to 30 days, with the exception of one hour after each meal (the magnet must stay off the stomach for one hour after meals in order for digestion to occur).

Other Treatment Options

Maladaptive reactions to foods are an important part of both acute and chronic diseases, including infections. Therefore, it is best to follow a Four-Day Diversified Rotation Diet to avoid these reactions. This diet involves the initial avoidance of any food that is used as often as twice per week. After three months, these foods can be reintroduced into the diet once again.

For the **Four-Day Diversified Rotation Diet**, see Appendix.

In addition, take oral supplements of vitamins C and E, selenium, taurine, cystine, glutathione, and coenzyme Q10, two or more hours prior to magnetic therapy. These oxygen regulators (antioxidants) can help eliminate free radicals produced by infectious microorganisms of any kind. A negative magnetic field is the strongest of antioxidants.

Inflammation

INFLAMMATION IS CHARACTERIZED by redness, swelling, pain, tenderness, heat, and disturbed function in a specific area of the body. Inflammatory reactions can occur in the joints, muscles, tendons, nerves, skin, brain, internal organs, or in any part of the human body.

Inflammation is often caused by acute maladaptive reactions to foods, chemicals, and inhalants. Acidity, which also produces a lack of oxygen (acid-hypoxia), is the common denominator of these maladaptive reactions, and they are usually accompanied by various types of discomfort and pain.

Treatment Options for Inflammation

Since maladaptive reactions to foods are often the major cause of inflammatory reactions, a Four-Day Diversified Rotation Diet—as well as a complete avoidance of all chemicals that produce symptoms—should be used to reduce inflammation. In addition, a thorough diagnostic and nutritional evaluation should be done, including an identification of any underlying illness. Magnetic therapy should be combined with other therapies that are specific for the demonstrated disease.

Inflammatory symptoms are the result of cellular edema (swelling), local acidity, and lack of oxygen. A negative magnetic field reverses these conditions, producing a normal, alkaline state with an abundance of molecular oxygen. This reverses inflammation and relieves the pain associated with it.

For the **Four-Day Diversified Rotation Diet**, see Appendix.

The negative magnetic field provides a normalization of the body's pH. It is also an energy activator of oxidoreductase enzymes, which free molecular oxygen from its bound state in free radicals, and raises the availability of molecular oxygen to inflamed areas of the body. This reduces inflammation and promotes healing in the body.

In order to treat inflammation, the negative magnetic field should be placed directly over the affected area. The size of the magnet should be larger than the area being treated. The higher the gauss strength of the magnet, the more effective the treatment. With magnetic pads, the plastiform magnets are cut into strips and placed close together in a nylon holder. As such, they are flexible and can be placed, without any pressure, across a breast, around a joint, and so forth. Ceramic magnets, such as the $1\frac{1}{2}$" x $\frac{1}{2}$" ceramic disc magnet, are excellent for many inflammatory areas, such as headaches or joint pain. The larger 4" x 6" x $\frac{1}{2}$" or 4" x 6" x 1" ceramic magnets are excellent for treating large joints, organs, or the spine. Acute inflammation and pain are usually relieved within ten to 30 minutes. It should be understood, however, that this type of magnetic treatment is not a nerve block, and some types of nerve pain will not be relieved.

It is a good practice to leave the magnets on the body even beyond the relief of pain, because it is valuable for reversing the disease process. When treating any type of inflammation, also use systemic treatment for the general improvement of the body, by sleeping with magnets at the crown of the head and on a negative magnetic field bed pad. The magnets in the bed pad are $1\frac{7}{8}$" x $\frac{7}{8}$" x $\frac{3}{8}$" mini-block magnets, placed $1\frac{1}{2}$" apart throughout the pad. People with generalized pains should sleep on this pad every night. At the crown of the head, four of the 4" x 6" x 1" ceramic magnets are placed $\frac{3}{4}$" apart in a wooden carrier held firmly against the headboard, and raised or lowered, depending on the height of the pillow. Keep the head as close as possible to the magnets.

Other systemic treatments include wearing a 5" x 6" double magnet, multi-magnet flexible mat over the heart (under the clothing) as much as possible. Placing two 1" x $\frac{1}{8}$" neodymium disc magnets over separate areas outside the clothing will hold the pad in place. This will magnetize the water and oxygen flowing through the heart, which will then circulate throughout the body. The negative magnetic field circulating through the body acts as a free-radical scavenger and an anti-inflammatory agent. When sitting down, sit on a comfort chair pad, which has magnets in the seat and the back. Organs, such as the liver, spleen, intestines, lungs, prostate, and vagina, should be treated with magnets that penetrate deeply into the body (for example, the 4" x 6" x $\frac{1}{2}$" ceramic magnets).

When treating specific inflamed areas of the body, choose an appropriate magnet. For example, inflamed lymph nodes should be treated with magnets of suitable size. Often, it is best to tape a 1" x ¹/₈" neodymium magnet directly over a small lymph node. However, if the lymph node is larger than one inch, a 1¹/₂" x ¹/₂" ceramic disc magnet (or plastiform magnets this size) should be used. The treatment should be continuous until the inflammation is completely gone.

Inflamed teeth and gums can be treated with either the ceramic disc or ceramic mini-block magnet. Tape the magnet on the face over the inflamed area at night. Initially, these magnets should be left on 24 hours a day for at least two weeks.

The 5" x 6" or 5" x 12" double magnet, multi-magnet pads are useful around joints; either can be reinforced with stronger magnets placed over inflamed areas. Flexible mats can be reinforced, if needed, by placing 1⁷/₈" x ⁷/₈" x ³/₈" mini-blocks on the positive pole side. Place the mini-blocks 1¹/₂" apart crosswise on the pad (three on the smaller mat, six on the larger mat). Plastiform magnets are available in 2", 3", and 4" widths, and as long a strip as needed; these may be bent around a joint (cover with duct tape to prevent the magnets from cracking).

Lupus

All lupus patients I have examined have been serious reactors to foods, especially cereal grains (wheat, rye, oats, and barley). The inflammatory symptoms of lupus often subside or even disappear with five days of avoidance of the commonly eaten foods. Furthermore, symptoms re-emerge as very painful inflammatory symptoms when the person eats gluten-bearing cereal grains. Therefore, it is important for

For the **Four-Day Diversified Rotation Diet**, see Appendix.

the lupus patient to always proceed with a Four-Day Diversified Rotation Diet.

Lupus is a systemic disease, with viruses (Epstein-Barr, cytomegalo, and human herpes #6) as the central causes. Treat systemically with a 70-magnet bed composed of 4"x 6" x 1" magnets placed 1" apart. Sleep all night on the bed and use for four 1-hour periods during the day. Minimum treatment time is three months.

In all inflammatory cases, it is also important to avoid the use of products that inhibit the production of melatonin and cause other more serious side effects. These include all tranquilizers, some antidepressants such as Prozac, alcohol, tobacco, caffeine, steroids, and non-steroidal, anti-inflammatory agents (such as aspirin, Tylenol, and Excedrin). Preferably, use magnets instead of drugs to relieve the symptoms of lupus, rheumatoid diseases, and other inflammatory diseases. If used skillfully, magnets are a better choice for symptom relief.

Hemorrhoids

Consider the possibility of food, chemical, and inhalant reactions as a factor in hemorrhoids. Also, drink enough water to ensure a loose stool. Sitting on the 4" x 6" x $\frac{1}{2}$" magnet has been very effective for treating hemorrhoids. Even bleeding hemorrhoids have responded well for some people. Sit on a comfort chair pad and slip the magnet under the rectal/genital area. Often, hemorrhoids are infected with bacteria, and thus are itchy; magnetic treatment can be very useful in handling these types of complications.

Men's Health Problems

NORMAL FUNCTION of the male genitourinary tract is essential to the overall health of a man's body. Because this system is susceptible to a number of conditions and disorders, special attention must be paid to its health in order to maintain healthy sexual function, proper elimination, and general vitality. The health of the genitourinary organs reflects a man's overall well-being. Some of the most common male health concerns include impotence and benign prostate problems.

Benign Prostatic Hypertrophy

By the age of 50, about 30% of all men will start to experience difficulties with urination related to enlargement of the prostate gland or benign prostatic hypertrophy (BPH). Increases in the number of times a man has to visit the bathroom along with a frequent sensation of having to urinate—especially at night—are among some of the early signs. In addition, a reduction in the force and caliber of urination is also characteristic of prostatic enlargement. Instability of the detrusor muscle (the outer muscle

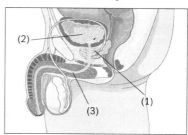

The prostate (1), a male sex gland, is located below the bladder (2) and encompasses the urethra (3). Typically in older men, the prostate tends to enlarge resulting in restricted urinary flow, bladder infections, or kidney damage.

layer of the bladder) can even result in urinary incontinence. These symptoms often lead to an increased sense of frustration and embarrassment, as well as the disruption of normal activities, translating into several billion dollars a year in related health management costs.

Enlargement of the prostate is usually caused by an abnormal overgrowth and/or swelling of the tissue of the prostate, which then blocks the urethra or opening from the bladder. Problems associated with this condition usually continue to worsen with age, increasing in incidence to about 50% of all males by the age of 60, and up to almost 80% past age 70.[1]

Magnet Therapy

Scott had to urinate five times each night due to a swollen prostate. A friend loaned him a 4" x 6" x ½" magnet. Scott put this magnet on a chair and sat on it for as many hours as he could during the day. Within one month, he was getting up to urinate only one time per night. Interestingly, Scott had a friend with the same problem, who used the same treatment. After one month of exposure, Scott's friend was also relieved of his difficulties.

Jim had a swollen prostate and was scheduled for surgery. For one month prior to surgery, Jim used the 4" x 6" x ½" magnet. When the physician examined Jim prior to surgery, he found no evidence of a swollen prostate and Jim did not have the surgery after all.

The usual magnetic treatment is to place a 5" x 12" double magnet, multi-magnet flexible mat across the lower abdomen with a 4" x 6" x ½" ceramic magnet lengthwise to the body directly over the center of this mat; apply for 24 hours a day. Hold in place with a 4" x 52" body wrap. When sitting, use a magnetic comfort chair pad with a 4" x 6" x ½" magnet under the seat.

Impotence

Impotence is defined as the inability to sustain a satisfactory erection to perform intercourse and ejaculation. It is estimated that about 10 million men in the United States are experiencing some form of impotence, of which only about 200,000 per year seek medical help.

Brief exposure of the genital area and gonads to the positive magnetic field has often been recommended to increase sex drive. This involves 15-30 minutes of exposure to the genital area, including the testes, to increase testosterone production as well as sexual drive. Unfortunately, the positive magnetic field will also encourage the growth of any existing viruses, bacteria, and fungi. It will also increase the growth of any existing prostate cancer, as well as further exaggerate an enlarged prostate. In light of these limitations, it is logical to discourage the use of a positive magnetic field.

On the other hand, the negative magnetic field is safe and effective. Sleep on a negative magnetic field bed pad with four 4" x 6" x 1" ceramic magnets at the crown of the head. This raises the general energy of the body and the sexual drive is a logical expression of this improved energy.

Nutritional Therapy

Vitamin C is a major component of the seminal vesicles and prostate gland, and high amounts are found in prostatic secretions. Vitamin E is also present and, due to its fat solubility, acts as an antioxidant and stabilizes membranes and lipids. Zinc has long been used in the treatment of the prostate, because of its prominent role in the metabolism of prostatic tissue as well as its sterilizing effect, which keeps the gland and urethra free of microorganisms.

A general vitamin and mineral supplementation routine is also beneficial, especially one high in B vitamins and magnesium. In numerous studies, magnesium has been shown to be an important nutrient that is deficient in most people.

Prevention

Prevention is the best approach to maintaining the health of the male organs. Following the Four-Day Diversified Rotation Diet with proper nutritional support is the best way to prevent prostate problems.

Caution: It is recommended by the American Cancer Society that males over the age of 40 receive yearly examinations for the presence of prostate enlargement and cancer. Reluctance to undergo examination on the part of many men often causes early treatment to be postponed, allowing the condition to become worse. It is only after symptoms become unbearable that many men seek treatment.

See "Male Health," pp. 733-743.

Early detection has become much simpler and more refined with the introduction of a few relatively noninvasive diagnostic procedures such as PSA (prostate specific antigen) blood testing, urinalysis, and ultrasound. Rectal ultrasound for visualization of the tumor is beneficial when used with these other tests. Because the procedure is relatively new, it is important that it be done by a physician experienced in the interpretation of ultrasound scans.

Mental and Emotional Problems

ANY DISTURBANCE in behavior, emotion, or cognition can be considered a form of mental disorder. Recent evidence suggests that depression, anxiety, antisocial behavior, learning disorders, or schizophrenia can be caused by biochemical imbalances, toxins, allergies, food sensitivities, and other environmental factors. According to the National Institute of Mental Health, over 28% of all Americans suffer from some type of mental disorder severe enough to require psychiatric treatment.[1] Incidences of depression and suicide are also rapidly increasing, especially among children and adolescents.

Types of Mental Disorders
Although there is no clear-cut way of defining mental disorders, they can be divided into several overlapping categories loosely defined as emotional, personality, and thought disorders.

Emotional Disorders—Two of the most common emotional disorders are depression and anxiety. Depression is characterized by feelings of persistent sadness, fear, unhappiness, pessimism, hopelessness, worthlessness, or despair. Serious depression, if not treated, can even lead to suicidal thoughts and feelings. Physiological symptoms may include a change in appetite (either increased or decreased), constipation, sleepiness, or sleeplessness.

Anxiety disorders, including phobias, affect roughly 10 million people,[2] with symptoms ranging from mild unease to intense fear and panic. These symptoms can often be manifested physically by tightness in the chest, hyperventilation, heart palpitations, or gastrointestinal problems.

Personality Disorders—Personality disorders are characterized by a person's inability to effectively relate socially, for a variety of reasons. People suffering from paranoia, for instance, are overly suspicious, narcissistic people tend to be selfish and self-centered, and antisocial people fail to conform to societal rules and regulations. Other personality disorders can include overdependence, insecurity, obsessiveness, compulsiveness, passiveness, and aggression. Patients with borderline personality disorders often have difficulty maintaining stable relationships and are often socially inappropriate and moody. Addictions such as those to alcohol, drugs, and gambling are also considered forms of personality disorders.

Thought Disorders—Thought disorders include conditions such as behavioral problems, learning difficulties, schizophrenia, dementia (confused thinking), delusions, and brain dysfunction. Manic and depressive behaviors can also be considered forms of thought disorders.

What Causes Mental Disorders?

Until recently, most mental disorders were considered either psychological in nature or genetically predisposed. Treatment options were generally limited to psychotherapy, or to medication, electroshock treatment, or surgical intervention. Today, however, many psychiatrists, psychologists, and researchers recognize that numerous factors can contribute to the onset of mental disorders, including social and cultural factors, age and gender, nutritional deficits, viral infections, allergies and food sensitivities, alcohol and drug addictions, and even prescription drugs, including those prescribed to treat mental illness.

Peter Breggin, M.D., a Harvard-trained psychiatrist, points out that drug therapy, while suppressing the symptoms of depression and other mental disorders, can also make a person chemically toxic, which will actually deepen the problem.[3] Illness can also be a major contributor to mental illness, as well as stress, both physical and emotional, chronic and acute. Exposure to environmental stresses from chemicals, toxins, and electromagnetic fields can also play a major role in one's mental health.

My clinical experience indicates that there is a common starting point for all organic brain disorders—a viral infection from the herpes family, namely, Epstein-Barr, cytomegallo, and human herpes virus #6. These infections occur during the gestation period in which the mother has a flare-up of infectious mononucleosis, herpes, or some other viral invasion related to these viruses. She then passes the infection on to the fetus. The infectious invasion into the child's brain can also occur in early childhood. As the child progresses through the early years of brain development, these viruses actually infect the neurons of the brain, producing a mild swelling within the brain. This swelling injures the developing brain, including the temporal lobe areas and especially the frontal part of the brain. When this occurs, perception, judgment, and the ability to concentrate are often severely damaged.

EDITOR'S NOTE
Drs. Philpott and Kalita have co-authored a book entitled *Brain Allergies: An Update* (NTC/ Contemporary Publishing, 2000), which contains additional information on the topics of maladaptive food, chemical, and inhalant reactions in relation to mental illness.

Studies reveal that Epstein-Barr, cytomegalo, and human herpes #6 viral infections are chronic and fluctuating, meaning they remain active in the body and brain, though they fluctuate in the severity of their symptomatic manifestation. As they grow in strength due to varying stresses within the child's life, these infections put additional stress on the immune system.

These are lymphotropic viruses that infect the immune system. B lymphocytes become disordered from the viral infection, producing antibodies and an autoimmiune response inappropriately. As a result, the child's immune system becomes compromised. The child becomes more reactive to chemicals and inhalants in the environment. This additional stress makes the child much more prone to maladaptively react to specific foods in the diet.

For example, schizophrenia is a state of disordered brain function in the areas of perception, mood, thought, and motor function. Acute mental symptoms can be triggered by maladaptive reactions to foods, chemicals, or inhalants to which the subject is allergic, addicted, or otherwise hypersensitive. Several studies have demonstrated that maladaptive reactions to environmental substances, especially foods, are significant factors in evoking mental illnesses.

From studying schizophrenia, I have concluded that its origin is the aforementioned viral infections. After being infected in the brain, the child often experiences learning difficulties or hyperactivity. Later on in adolescence or in the early twenties, the person develops full-blown schizophrenia, manic-depressive reactions, or psychotic depression. All suffer from maladaptive reactions and also have multiple and often severe nutritional deficiencies.

Schizophrenics also have chronic, abnormally high electrical discharges from deep within the brain, especially from the amygdala or the mid-temporal area of the right and left hemispheres. Post-mortem studies show that schizophrenics have higher than normal amounts of dopamine (a neurotransmitter) in the amygdala.

Many psychological disorders are caused by electromagnetic imbalances in the body. Anxieties, phobias, obsessions, compulsions, depression, psychosis, and seizures evoke an abnormal rise in the electrical activity of the central nervous system. Such conditions can be controlled with negative magnetic energy, eliminating or reducing the severity of the disorder.

Success Story: Psychotic Depression

Gerald, a sociology professor, developed a psychotic depression. He would not drink or eat. Tranquilizers and antidepressants did not change his symptoms. After six weeks in the hospital, his wife was informed that the only therapy left with potential value was electric shock treatment (EST). She declined EST and asked me to take him as a patient.

I told his psychiatrist that EST produced a magnetic anesthesia which would be helpful, but that there was also a magnetic treatment without the side effects of EST. Gerald reclined on a massage table covered with 4" x 6" x ½" magnets; under his head was a stack of eight 4" x 6" x ½" magnets. Gerald also had an intravenous solution for hydration and nutrients, containing vitamins C and B6, calcium, and magnesium. He was asleep within five minutes. With the properly administered magnetic treatment, Gerald's psychotic depression was reversed in one hour. It would have taken a dozen or more electric shock treatments to achieve this same goal, and there would more than likely be at least temporary memory loss associated with EST.

Success Story: Psychosis

Cindy, a teenage girl with schizo-affective psychosis, as well as a history of depression with social withdrawal, irritability, headache, confusion, and gastric upset, had attempted suicide. Her parents reported that these major symptoms would last up to four days after she ate gluten-containing grains (wheat, rye, oats, and barley).

She fasted on water only for five days, by which time she was symptom-free. After the fifth day, she reacted to wheat with symptoms of withdrawal, depression, and headache. Then, we placed the negative pole of a 4" x 12" x ⅛" strip magnet down her spine and placed the negative pole of ceramic disc magnets bitemporally. Within five minutes, she was asleep and she slept for 45 minutes. When Cindy woke up, she was completely symptom-free.

A few days later, we repeated the procedure for 30 minutes before she ate a meal of a reactive food. She experienced no symptoms this time. We could relieve the symptoms of a known maladaptive food and also prevent the symptoms from developing by treating her ahead of time. She continues to do well by maintaining her rotation diet.

Success Story: Autism

At 5, Tim was correctly diagnosed as autistic. Since both his parents were physicians, he was given every therapeutic, medical, and educational opportunity possible. By age 17, he was schizophrenic. He could only speak in grunts accompanied by bizarre facial and arm movements. He was covered with acne from head to foot, and no antibiotic seemed to help.

Episodically, he had periods of saying the word "circle" at three-second intervals. With the placement of the negative pole of a 4" x 6" x $1/2$" magnet on the back of his head and upper neck, he would stop his compulsive verbalization. His acne cleared on the withdrawal from his frequently eaten foods and emerged again with a test meal of cow's milk, showing a maladaptive reaction.

With behavioral training and temporally placed magnets used to hold symptoms in abeyance, Tim was taught to speak clearly without his former bizarre facial and arm gesturing. He was also taught to drive a car and even attended a university as a special student in the art department. The mental symptoms of patients like Tim can routinely be reversed by the elimination of maladaptive foods and chemicals. Symptoms that do by chance develop during treatment are quickly eliminated by magnetic therapy. Ninety-five percent of symptom-producing foods can be returned to the rotation diet after three months, without provoking symptoms.

Treatment Options for Mental Illnesses

The treatment goal for mental illnesses is, first and foremost, to eliminate all food, chemical, and inhalant maladaptive reactions, and improve nutritional status. It is also important to calm the electrical activity and excessive dopamine production in the brain. In order to accomplish this, simultaneous placement of a negative magnetic field on the right and left temporal areas provides maximum control. Usually, most mental symptoms can be controlled within ten minutes by using ceramic or neodymium disc magnets in this manner.

In the field of psychiatry, magnetic therapy is replacing electroconvulsive therapy for depression and other major mental disorders. In addition, magnetic therapy is replacing tranquilizers, antidepressants and anti-seizure medications in the treatment of major mental disorders. Anxiety, tension, depression, obsessions and compulsions can be alleviated with a negative magnetic field application to the brain.

Magnet Therapy

All those with mental illnesses should sleep on a magnetic bed pad, composed of $1^{7}/_{8}$" x $^{7}/_{8}$" x $^{3}/_{8}$" mini-block magnets placed $1^{1}/_{2}$" apart. Also, place magnets at the crown of the head (four 4" x 6" x 1" magnets placed $^{3}/_{4}$" apart). These can be raised or lowered, depending on the height of the pillow, with the top of the head as close as possible to the magnets.

At night, sleep with a 5" x 12" double magnet, multi-magnet flexible mat crosswise on the lower abdomen. In the center of this mat, place a 4" x 6" x $^{1}/_{2}$" magnet lengthwise on the body, held in place with a 4" x 52" body wrap. This placement will help rid the body of any viral, fungal, or parasitic infections anywhere in the pelvic area. It will also stimulate the intestinal wall to produce melatonin, an important hormone for sleep and mood.[4] At night, place a 5" x 12" double magnet, multi-magnet flexible mat, with six mini-blocks $1^{1}/_{2}$" apart on the positive pole side, over the front of the chest; hold in place with a 4" x 52" body wrap. This treats the heart, lungs, thymus gland, and, in women, the breasts.

It is important to treat the heart with magnets because the water and oxygen flowing through the heart will be magnetized and carried to the entire body. Also, when sitting down, use a comfort chair pad with magnets in the seat and back.

For treating most mental symptoms, use the $1^{1}/_{2}$" x $^{1}/_{2}$" ceramic disc magnets; a headband can align the magnets bitemporally. This treatment usually requires about ten minutes to relieve major symptoms, but the more hours of negative field magnetic exposure, the better.

■ For obsessive-compulsiveness, place a 4" x 6" x $^{1}/_{2}$" ceramic magnet on the back of the head. An alternative is to place a 4" x 6" x $^{1}/_{8}$" plastiform magnet directly over the occiput (base of the cranium at the back of the head), with a neodymium disc magnet over the center, as well as a ceramic disc on the left temporal area.

■ For anxieties and phobias, place a $1^{1}/_{2}$" x $^{1}/_{2}$" ceramic disc magnet on the left temporal area and another on the forehead. A negative magnetic field applied to the forehead encourages relaxation, increases alertness, and improves memory. The usual treatment is bitemporal placement (just above and in front of the ears) of $1^{1}/_{2}$" x $^{1}/_{2}$" ceramic disc magnets, held in place with a 2" x 26" headband. This treatment is also effective for tension, depression, and obsessions.

■ Depression, delusions, and hallucinations are usually best handled with bitemporal placement of ceramic disc magnets. Centered in the temporal areas of the head are the amygdala; treating the amygdala can calm down the entire brain.

Diet and Nutrition

The most important factor involved in any mental symptom-reduction plan is the strict avoidance of maladaptive reactions to chemicals, inhalants, and especially foods. The Four-Day Diversified Rotation Diet, combined with an initial three months of complete avoidance of reactive substances, does much to relieve symptoms of all mental disorders. The rotation diet is to be a lifestyle. It is also important for the person to avoid using tobacco, alcohol, caffeine, or any other addictive substance. Furthermore, clinical testing of the patient's nutritional status should be done and nutritional deficiencies corrected immediately.

For those with mental disorders, a laboratory analysis for levels of vitamins, minerals, and amino acids, as well as antibodies to viruses and toxic metals should be done. I have seen thousands of patients with mental disorders and they are routinely infected with one or more lymphotropic viruses (Epstein-Barr, cytomegalo, and human herpes #6), which injure the brain. Maladaptive food reactions evoke symptoms because the brain has first been injured by a viral infection.

Oxidoreductase enzymes are necessary for energy production and for processing the by-products of oxidation (free radicals, peroxides, oxyacids, alcohols, and aldehydes) and toxins produced by microorganisms. Nutrition is important for enzyme function, because they are composed of amino acids, vitamins (especially B complex), and minerals. However, nutritional therapy, such as mega-vitamins, ignores an important fact—a negative magnetic field is an energy activator of these enzymes. Symptoms can be routinely and predictably reversed with exposure to a negative magnetic field, even with demonstrable nutritional deficiencies.

To treat the viral infections, sleep on a 70-magnet bed of 4" x 6" x 1" ceramic block magnets placed 1" apart. Sleep on the bed through the night and for four 1-hour periods during the day. Allow at least three months for treatment.

For the **Four-Day Diversified Rotation Diet**, see Appendix.

Multiple Sclerosis

NEARLY 350,000 AMERICANS are affected by one of medicine's most misunderstood diseases, multiple sclerosis. Often, the early detection and identification of underlying causes combined with strict dietary and lifestyle guidelines can stabilize or reverse the symptoms.

Multiple sclerosis (MS) is a disease of the central nervous system and usually occurs in early adult life. MS is often marked by numbness, loss of balance, clumsiness, sensitivity to heat and cold, blurred or double vision, feelings of pins and needles in the hands and feet, and difficulty walking. In advanced stages of MS, walking becomes more difficult, movements become more spastic, arms and hands may become extremely weak, speech can become slurred, and chronic urinary urgency or incontinence may develop. Fatigue, one of the "silent" and most disabling symptoms of MS, may render even the smallest tasks difficult.

Multiple sclerosis involves the myelin surrounding the neurons of the central nervous system (CNS). In such a scenario, the myelin swells, which puts pressure on the neurons, and this pressure inhibits their proper function. This process is termed *extinction of disuse*. Fortunately, however, the MS disease process does not kill a sizable number of neurons. Since most of the neurons are still alive, their function can be reinstated after the acute swelling of the myelin has been reduced.

What Causes Multiple Sclerosis?

By the time multiple sclerosis is actually diagnosed—usually in a person's twenties or thirties—the disease is well established, having taken root in either adolescence or childhood. MS is caused by an infection of the human herpes virus #6, which is consistently present in those with MS.[1]

Intolerance to foods frequently eaten by the MS sufferer is also a routine finding. While these intolerances are not the cause of MS, they can further irritate the virus-damaged central nervous system. A Four-Day Diversified Rotation Diet is thus essential in managing MS.

Reactions to environmental toxins can also precipitate symptoms in MS, because of viral damage to the nervous system. Mercury is a highly toxic metal that, when used in dental amalgam fillings, can seep into body tissues where it accumulates and becomes capable of producing symptoms in the body that are indistinguishable from those of MS.[2]

For the **Four-Day Diversified Rotation Diet**, see Appendix.

According to Hal Huggins, D.D.S., of Colorado Springs, Colorado, mercury poisoning often remains undetected because a patients' symptoms do not necessarily suggest mercury as the initiating cause, but the effects of mercury toxicity are potentially devastating. Mercury has been recognized as a poison since the 1500s, yet mercury amalgams have been used in dentistry since the 1820s.

Mercury has been shown to bind to the DNA of cells and cell membranes, causing cell distortion and inhibited cell function.[3] When this happens the immune system no longer recognizes the cell as part of the body and initiates an autoimmune reaction, destroying myelin in the process. MS patients have been found to have over seven times higher levels of mercury in their cerebrospinal fluid (the fluid that surrounds the brain and spinal cord) as compared to neurologically healthy patients.[4]

Mercury toxicity is damaging, but does not initiate the myelin damage in MS. Nevertheless, sources of mercury should be removed from the body for general health reasons.

Treatment Options for Multiple Sclerosis

Maladaptive reactions to foods are generally not the initiating cause of multiple sclerosis, but these food maladaptive reactions become a serious part of the illness. More specifically, the central nervous system becomes a target tissue for these reactions, triggering more severe MS symptoms. The Four-Day Diversified Rotation Diet can

For the **Four-Day Diversified Rotation Diet**, see Appendix.

help prevent these damaging food reactions. This diet involves the initial avoidance of frequently used symptom-producing foods, as well as subsequent reintroduction of foods on a rotation basis.

Magnet Therapy

Magnetic therapy can aid in the correction of three specific problem areas related to MS: the need to eliminate viral infections, reducing the swelling of myelin, and reinstating central nervous system function. Initial treatment is sleeping on a super magnetic bed during the night and for four 1-hour periods during the day, for a period of three months. The magnetic bed is composed of 70 4" x 6" x 1" ceramic block magnets placed 1" apart.

After the initial three-month magnetic treatment, it is time to attempt to reinstate neuron function, which consists of practice sessions using a positive magnetic field. A 4" x 24" plastiform magnet or a 5" x 12" double magnet, multi-magnet flexible mat used on the spine is turned over to the positive field side and applied for a period of three minutes. The person exercises the arms and legs to reinstate function. When the three minutes are over, the magnet is turned over to the negative field side and is applied for a five-minute period. Again, the person exercises the arms and legs. Repeat several times during any given practice session. Afterwards, maintain a negative magnetic field exposure for at least 30 minutes.

The positive magnetic field can also be used to reinstate brain function. Apply the positive field side of a 4" x 6" x ½" magnet on the side, front, or back of the head for a three-minute period only. Practice functional exercises (eye exercises as well as performance in speech, reading, and comprehension) during these three minutes. Then, apply the negative magnetic field for a five-minute period. Switch back and forth several times for a total practice session of 15-20 minutes.

Biological Dentistry

The removal of mercury-containing dental fillings is an intrinsic part of the treatment for any degenerative disease, including multiple sclerosis. According to Dr. Huggins, mercury vapor escaping from dental fillings can interfere with the action of key enzymes, thus disturbing important enzymatic functions in the body. He adds that mercury vapor is implicated in chronic fatigue, a common MS symptom.

Replacing mercury fillings with other kinds of material, however, is not as straightforward as it seems. Dr. Huggins warns that some plastic materials can contain aluminum and thereby create different problems for the patient. Before any work is begun, patients of Dr. Huggins first receive a "bio-compatibility blood test" to determine which alternative material is biologically compatible.

Dr. Huggins explains, "Patient blood serum is tested against multiple dental materials. Some dental materials cause immune reactions and others immune suppression. Neither are healthy conditions. An example of overreactivity is multiple sclerosis, and of immune suppression is AIDS. Since no material is 100% safe any more than no one prescription drug is safe for everyone, we do immunologic testing on each patient's blood to determine where reactivity is. After identifying the high and minimal reactivities, a computer matches dental materials with reactivity and suggests the safest materials for that particular patient."

Hyperbaric Oxygen Therapy

In hyperbaric oxygen therapy (HBOT), a patient is placed in an oxygen chamber. Atmospheric pressure is then elevated in order to increase the amount of oxygen entering the body's tissues. As well as oxygenating the tissues, HBOT may also enhance the immune sys-

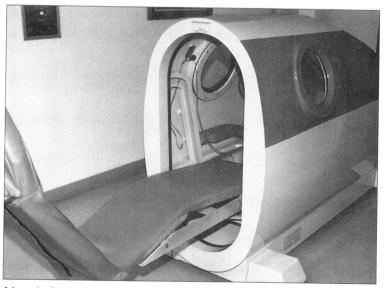

A hyperbaric oxygen chamber, somewhat resembling a miniature submarine, delivers pure oxygen under pressure to all the cells of the body, including the brain.

See "Oxygen Therapy," pp. 412-421.

tem, reduce inflammation via its effects on prostaglandins, help in the repair of damaged blood vessels, stimulate the circulation in the small blood vessels, and, in a variety of ways, assist in the production of myelin. Bladder and bowel dysfunction are two of the symptoms of multiple sclerosis which most improve with HBOT.[5]

Exactly how this procedure works for patients with MS is still a matter of conjecture and debate. While some medical literature refutes HBOT's effectiveness, in Britain, several thousand people with MS have received HBOT treatments. From 1983 to 1987, 500,000 individual sessions were provided, and nearly half of the 4,000 people involved benefited in one or more ways.[6] HBOT seems to have been effective in keeping many people from getting worse, often improving their general condition and reversing many minor symptoms.

Although HBOT has an established value in treating MS, it is not as oxygenating as the super magnetic bed.

Obesity

THE UNMISTAKABLE FACT is that Americans are getting fatter. According to statistics from the National Institutes of Health, 33% of American adults are considered obese. This number is up from 25% of adults in 1980, a significant increase in such a short period of time,[1] which works out to an average weight gain of eight pounds per person.[2] The overweight problem continues with our children as well. The U.S. Centers for Disease Control (CDC) estimates that 21% of children between the ages of 12 and 19 are overweight, up from 15% in the late 1970s.[3] Children who have overweight parents tend to be overweight themselves, and overweight children tend to have weight problems as adults.[4]

We are growing more and more overweight even as we obsess about our appearance and particularly about staying thin. But this isn't just a matter of appearances: obesity (weight that is 20% above normal for your height) is thought to contribute to a wide range of other health problems, including diabetes, heart disease, and cancer. The health costs associated with obesity are staggering, according to researchers at Harvard University. Obesity is a factor in 19% of the cases of heart disease, with annual health costs estimated at almost $30 billion; 57% of adult-onset diabetes cases ($9 billion); 10% of cases of musculoskeletal disease ($3.75 billion); 30% of gallbladder disease ($3.2 billion); and 23% of cancer cases ($0.67 billion).[5] Obesity may be a contributing factor in as many as 300,000 deaths each year.[6]

What Causes Obesity?

What causes weight gain is pretty straightforward: you consume more calories from food than the body uses or burns off in its daily tasks. The person with a weight problem must take responsibility for their eating habits and for correcting the situation. Keep in mind that food addictions are a factor in obesity and obsessive-compulsiveness about food. With addictions, there is a relief of symptoms on initial contact with the addictive substance, for instance, a favorite food. This releases endorphins and other body-produced pain-killers that alleviate symptoms. When these endorphins again reach a low level, the person again reaches for the addictive food, leading to a seesaw effect of addiction and relief. This process is a factor in obesity.

Whether or not a person becomes obese depends on a number of factors, including genetics, societal influences, amount of physical activity, and psychological makeup.[7]

■ Researchers have found that obesity tends to run in families. This may be partially due to genetics, but could also be influenced by dietary and lifestyle habits learned as a child, including the kinds of food you tend to eat (for example, high-fat or processed foods) and how often you eat.

■ We're exercising too little: the amount of exercise you get on a regular basis will strongly affect your weight. Our lives in general are less physically active than for previous generations and most of us aren't getting enough exercise to make up for it. Children in America now spend an estimated two-and-a-half hours per day watching television.[8] A quarter of the population is completely sedentary while 55% are "inadequately active" according to the CDC.[9]

■ Perhaps, living in the "consumer culture" of United States, it is our just reward to be consuming ourselves to death. Not only are we eating more, but the kinds of foods we consume—fast foods, processed and high in fat—offer the least nutrition and the most potential for adding fat to our hips. And we're eating too much, period: average calorie intake is over 2,000 calories per day compared to 1,800 calories in the 1970s.[10] The food industry is doing its part to keep us "living large"—it spends $36 billion every year on advertising and a typical child sees up to 10,000 food commercials every year.[11]

■ Psychology may play a significant role in weight gain: many people who overeat do so in response to stress, anger, sadness, boredom, or other emotional factors unrelated to hunger or nutritional needs.[12] Foods affect moods by triggering the release of endorphins, the body's natural pain-killers, and the brain chemical serotonin, a mood regulator. Unfortunately, these foods (chocolate, carbohydrates, sweets) not only elevate your mood but also trigger cravings for more.[13] This kind of "emotional eating" can contribute significantly to weight gain if you lead a stressful life or have unresolved emotional issues.

■ In addition, many practitioners look for underlying imbalances that may contribute to weight gain, including an underactive thyroid, hormone imbalances, food allergies, yeast infections, and parasites.

Treatment Options for Obesity

Reduced caloric intake is the key answer for obesity. Magnet therapy can overcome the eating obsessions that come with food addictions. During a compulsive urge, place $1^{1}/_{2}$" x $^{1}/_{2}$" ceramic discs bitemporally, using a 2" x 26" band to hold in place. Postpone acting on the urges for 5-10 minutes while the negative magnetic field calms the brain. Some people may need to use a left temporal and low occipital (back of the skull) placement. Withdrawal symptoms can be managed by placing a 4" x 6" x $^{1}/_{2}$" magnet over the symptom area.

All addictions must be stopped at the same time, including tobacco, alcohol, drugs, and foods. Fast on water only, watermelon, or a single, seldom-used food for five days. Keep the body alkalinized by taking $^{1}/_{2}$ tsp to 1 tsp of sodium bicarbonate, 2-3 times per day, during the fast. After the fast, food testing can be done to determine symptom-producing foods. Then use the Four-Day Diversified Rotation Diet as a lifestyle.

When exposed to a negative magnetic field, fat deposits slowly regress over the course of several weeks. The most significant area for fat reduction is the abdomen; this area will reduce in size after placing a suitable magnet across the abdomen while asleep. For example, Arthur weighed 185 pounds. He placed two 4" x 6" x $^{1}/_{2}$" magnets two inches apart on his abdomen. Two weeks later, he had lost ten pounds, without making any dietary changes.

In order to obtain these weight-loss results, a magnet of suitable size needs to be placed directly over the abdomen. This magnet can be one 4" x 12" plastiform magnet or two of these can be fastened together. Hold in place with a 4" x 52" body wrap.

For more on **strategies for weight loss**, see *Weight Loss: An Alternative Medicine Definitive Guide* (AlternativeMedicine. com Books, 2000; ISBN 1-887299-19-X); to order, call 800-333-HEAL.

You may also choose to sleep with the double magnet, multi-magnet flexible mat across the abdomen or the 11" x 17" multipurpose pad. It is important to treat fat deposits at night while there is sufficient growth hormone to burn the fat. Human growth hormone (HGH) is released mostly at night. One of the functions of HGH is to metabolize fat, which requires enzymes and a negative magnetic field to

For the **Four-Day Diversified Rotation Diet**, see Appendix.

provide the energy for this action. Treat any area of the body that needs fat reduction. At this point, there are no statistical studies supporting the magnetic reduction of fat and only a few anecdotal cases. However, this magnetic fat-reducing theory should be investigated further.

Exercise

Food fuels the furnace of metabolism; exercise stokes its fire. Yet, almost as important as exercise, is what kind of exercise one does. Exercise that causes sweating and heavy breathing is sugar-burning exercise. Overweight people need fat-burning exercise, which requires slow, sustained activity. Practitioners generally recommend 45-60 minutes of vigorous walking every day, if possible. Exercise such as walking possesses many health benefits including increasing the metabolic rate.[14] An infrared sauna is ideal for burning calories. The key is finding an activity one likes and then changing exercise plans periodically to alleviate boredom.

Pain and Injuries

CHRONIC PAIN HAS BECOME the most common health disorder in the U.S., affecting nearly one out of three Americans, and costing nearly $40 billion a year in medical bills and lost wages.[1] Today, many therapies are available which have proven effective at both reducing chronic pain symptoms and alleviating their causes. Self-help methods can also be utilized, thus reducing the cost of treating chronic pain as well.

Everyone has experienced pain at some point in their life—a person stubs a toe and feels pain, a person is injured in an accident and feels pain. Yet, for some types of pain, there seems to be no underlying reason. It is just there, every day, interfering with one's daily pursuits and the enjoyment of life. This type of pain is categorized as chronic pain.

Pain can be caused by traumatic nerve energy, but most pain is caused by cellular swelling or edema, which leads to higher acidity in the body. Tissues with high levels of acid are painful, regardless of the initial cause. Toxins in the body accumulate because acidity blocks the enzymes that would normally eliminate them. While a negative magnetic field does not work well in relieving pain due to nerve injuries (it is not a nerve block), it is excellent for the more common pain due to acid-hypoxia.

The Magnetic Aspects of Pain

Robert O. Becker, M.D., an orthopedic surgeon and researcher in magnetics, discovered significant facts about bone injuries. For instance, he demonstrated that when a bone is injured, the area of injury initially registers electromagnetic positive. When an injury occurs, the body sends an electromagnetic positive signal of alarm to the brain through the nervous system and the brain returns an electromagnetic negative message to the site of injury through the cells that surround the nerves. As a result, when an injury occurs, the injury site initially contains a positive magnetic field that signals pain.[2]

Pain, which can be acute, intermittent, or chronic, is the body's most obvious signal of injury. Bruises, cuts, snake or insect bites, toxic substances, metabolic by-products of microorganisms, and maladaptive reactions to foods, chemicals, and inhalants all produce pain.

Swollen cells (caused by toxins, particularly acids which are often a result of injury) lead to the most pain. An acid state accompanies all injuries and simultaneously produces swollen cells. A deficiency of oxygen is also associated with high acidity. Acidity, lack of oxygen, and swollen cells thus make up the unpleasant picture of pain.

When we experience the pain of a broken bone, we do many things to hold the two broken bones together and relieve the pain. However, these efforts at healing would be useless unless there was also an electromagnetic energy field that simultaneously began the healing process of the broken bone.

A few hours after a bone is broken, the body begins to concentrate a negative magnetic field at the injury site. This is true of any injury—broken bone, cut, bruise, abrasion, or maladaptive reaction. It is the negative magnetic field that begins the healing process at a specific site of injury, and without it there would be no healing.

Thus, a positive magnetic field is the signal of inflammation, pain, and injury, which registers both locally and in the brain. On the other hand, the electromagnetic negative field of energy must be maintained in order for pain to subside and injuries to heal. A negative magnetic field is needed to govern all components of the healing process: reducing pain, inflammation, and edema; normalizing the local pH; and activating oxidoreductase enzymes, which neutralize free radicals and release molecular oxygen.

As a result, the negative magnetic field inhibits infectious microorganisms, eliminates toxins, relieves inflammation and edema, and facilitates cellular repairs. It floods the injured areas with oxygen and stimulates the production of melatonin and growth hormone. In order to supplement the body's own negative field of energy, a negative magnetic field from a static field magnet can be used over any fracture, skin cut, bruise, or injury site.

For more about **magnet therapy and inflammation**, see Inflammation. For more about **magnet therapy for infections**, see Infections.

Success Stories: Magnets for Pain Relief

Alan, a male in his fifties, suffered multiple injuries in an accident. He had constant pain in various parts of his body for several years. He underwent an MRI test and discovered that, for several hours afterward, he was free of pain. Based on this evidence, he purchased a negative magnetic field bed pad. After sleeping on this pad at night, his pain disappeared. He remained free of pain thereafter as long as he slept on a magnetic bed pad.

Tom, 60, was experiencing pain from diabetic neuropathy in both legs. He obtained relief in just 15 minutes by placing the negative field of a 4" x 6" x $^1/_2$" magnet on the painful areas. Periodic magnetic treatment maintained pain relief and he was able to sleep again at night, which he had not been able to do for a long time.

Sarah suffered from severe pain in her left hip. She was unable to take any drugs without life-threatening reactions. Instead, she placed a 4" x 6" ceramic magnet underneath her left hip as well as a mat over the top and side of the area. She gained considerable relief from this magnetic treatment within a short period of time.

Jane, a woman in her fifties, had an inoperable, ruptured lumbar disc. She was experiencing chronic pain and was unable to lift any appreciable weight. After sleeping on a negative magnetic bed pad for eight months, her pain was gone. X rays showed complete healing of the ruptured disc.

Marsha, 56, inadvertently punctured the knuckle of her right ring finger. She used two ceramic magnets to treat this deep wound, keeping the magnets over the wound for most of the day. Every time she would try to remove them, her finger would begin to swell and turn red. The next day, she put the magnets on the finger in the morning and removed them in the early evening; by then, the wound had completely healed.

David, 39, would periodically experience searing pain from his elbow to his wrist, keeping him awake at night. He had sustained an injury to his elbow while racing motorcycles in his youth. He applied the negative field of a 4" x 6" x $^1/_2$" ceramic magnet to his injured elbow and the pain subsided.

Treatment Options for Pain and Injuries

Much as a cut heals and a broken bone mends without any external help, the body has made a provision for pain to be eased by natural means such as the production of endorphins, an analgesic hormone which can produce euphoric and painkilling effects when released. Rather than just suppressing the symptoms of pain, as drug therapy does, doctors and pain therapists using magnet therapy utilize and activate these natural healing properties of the body.

Diet and Nutrition

According to James Braly, M.D., Medical Director of Immuno Labs, in Fort Lauderdale, Florida, diet and nutrition can both play important roles in the treatment of chronic pain. "I have seen patients who have tried just about everything to relieve their pain, only to finally find relief when they made changes in their diet and added supplements with proven pain-relieving properties," he says. Dr. Braly points out that inflammation, one of the principle mechanisms related to chronic pain, is often caused by an allergic reaction. "Often the reactions are due to food allergies," Dr. Braly notes. "If chronic pain symptoms seem to have no other discernible cause, testing for food allergies is advisable."

For the **Four-Day Diversified Rotation Diet**, see Appendix.

Once the maladaptive foods have been determined, they should be completely eliminated from the diet for a minimum of three months. After that, they can be reintroduced as part of a rotation diet, with no one food being eaten more than once in any four-day period. Dr. Braly also recommends limiting foods high in saturated fats, including red meats, dairy products, warm-water shellfish, partially hydrogenated oils, as well as avoiding alcohol and severely limiting caffeine.

He suggests a diet high in fiber and nonallergenic complex carbohydrates. "Organic, free-range poultry, cold sea-water fish, and sources of vegetable protein are also good," he says, "while margarine, shortenings, and other sources of partially hydrogenated oils should be omitted. Simple or refined sugars, including fruit juices, sodas, and pastries, are also culprits."

Along with diet, Dr. Braly suggests the following nutritional supplements be taken daily when in pain: vitamin C to 90% of bowel tolerance; evening primrose oil, which supplies essential fatty acids to reduce inflammation and decrease pain; vitamin E; and magnesium glycinate.

Magnet Therapy

Applying a negative magnetic field is highly effective in treating both the symptoms and causes of pain. Rather than just suppressing the symptoms of pain, as drug therapy does, the application of a negative magnetic field activates its internal healing mechanisms and supports and supplements your body's effort to repair its painful injuries.

Magnetic field therapy has many applications for the relief of pain. The negative magnetic field is ideal for relieving pain due to its ability to quickly normalize the metabolic functions that create the conditions in the first place. The negative magnetic field does not act as a painkiller, or analgesic, but as a normalizer of disordered metabolism.

When treating injuries and pain, one goal of magnetic treatment is to magnetize the entire body with a negative magnetic field. This maximizes the production of melatonin[3] and growth hormone (SEE QUICK DEFINITION), increases the levels of molecular oxygen, and alkalinizes the body's pH. In this way, magnetic therapy will optimize the healing of injuries and reduce pain faster and more efficiently.

Magnets relieve pain in two ways:

■ By evoking the production of endorphins in the body with the stress of a positive magnetic field. Raising endorphins can relieve pain, but the positive magnetic field also stimulates microorganisms and cancer growth. In fact, the positive magnetic field actually blocks the healing process and, for this reason, should not be used (alone or combined with a negative field).

■ A negative magnetic field replaces the acidity and low oxygen causing the pain with alkalinity and high oxygen, which relieves the pain. This also blocks the growth of microorganisms and cancer. This method is recommended over the use of a positive magnetic field.

Sleep on a magnetic bed pad ($1^7/_8$" x $^7/_8$" x $^3/_8$" mini-block magnets placed $1^1/_2$" apart) to expose the entire body. Treating the abdomen will stimulate the intestinal tract to produce melatonin. In addition to having magnets on

QUICK DEFINITION

Melatonin, a hormone produced by the pea-sized, light-sensitive pineal (pronounced pie-NEEL) gland in the center of the brain, regulates the body's internal clock, or circadian rhythm, which determines the 24-hour sleep-wake cycle. With aging, the peak in melatonin secretion is about one hour later than normal (normal peak secretion time is about 2 a.m.), and the maximum peak of melatonin is only one-half the level of young adults. Low melatonin levels have been associated with sleeping disturbances and light-related conditions such as seasonal affective disorder (SAD). Eating vitamin- and mineral-rich foods and increasing your exposure to bright light can improve the body's natural melatonin production.

Human growth hormone (HGH), naturally secreted by the pituitary gland in the brain, is a small, protein-like hormone similar to insulin. HGH is secreted in very brief pulses during the early hours of sleep and remains in circulation for only a few minutes. During adolescence, when growth is most rapid, production of HGH is high. After age 20, HGH production declines progressively at an average rate of about 14% per decade; by age 60, it is not uncommon to measure a growth hormone loss of 75% or more. In the early 1980s, growth hormone extracts were used to correct disturbances in normal growth; later it was synthesized for adult use. Benefits from HGH include increased muscle mass; improved physical strength; reduced fatigue; decreased fat (especially abdominal fat); increased bone strength; revitalization of liver, kidney, spleen, and brain functions; increased exercise capacity; strong kidney blood flow and efficiency; improved cardiac function; reduced risk from cardiovascular problems; and a general enhancement in the sense of well-being.

the mattress, it is useful to have a negative magnetic field at the top of the head, using a wooden carrier that holds magnets against the head-board (four 6" x 4" x 1" ceramic magnets are placed $^3/_4$" apart in the carrier). The magnets can be raised or lowered, depending upon the height of the pillow. The top of the head should be as close as possible to these magnets in order to provide deep, sound, energy-restoring sleep, and stimulate melatonin production by the pineal gland.

Local Magnetic Treatment

Arms and Legs—If injured, the long bones of the upper and lower arms and legs should be treated with magnets of sufficient length and width to cover the break. A bone that is fractured (with or without separation) should be treated under medical supervision with the usual bracing. A magnet can be placed on the outside of this brace, as the magnetic field can penetrate through a cast. Use a 2" x 5" x $^1/_2$" magnet, placed on one side of the limb. The negative field should always face the body.

On larger areas, such as the upper or lower leg, the 4" x 6" x $^1/_2$" magnet is preferable. Or you can wrap a 5" x 12" double magnet, multi-magnet flexible mat down the limb and then place the 2" x 5" x $^1/_2$" or the 4" x 6" x $^1/_2$" ceramic magnet on top of this mat. For bone breaks, magnetic application should be extended well past the complete healing stage. Magnetic treatment will speed up the healing time and should be maintained as continuously as possible, with removal only for brief, required periods, such as taking a bath.

Fingers and Toes—The long bones and joints of the fingers and hands must be treated with a magnet that adequately covers the entire area. A single break in a small bone may be bridged properly with either a $1^1/_2$" x $^1/_2$" ceramic disc magnet or a $1^7/_8$" x $^7/_8$" x $^3/_8$" mini-block magnet. An entire hand can be wrapped in a 5" x 6" or 5" x 12" double magnet, multi-magnet flexible mat. Even in this case, treat the local area with a suitable disc or mini-block magnet. These magnets can be taped directly over the break and held in place with an elastic wrap. Arthritic finger joints can be treated with the 1" x $^1/_8$" neodymium disc magnet, bound directly over the joint. Another suitable magnet is the $1^7/_8$" x $^7/_8$" x $^3/_8$" mini-block magnet. Toe joints can be treated in the same manner.

Ankles—Wrap the ankle in a 5" x 6" or 5" x 12" double magnet, multi-magnet flexible mat. The long bones of the foot and toes can be treated with a ceramic disc or the mini-block magnets. Bruised bones produce bone spikes in the heels, which can be treated with a disc magnet. Treat as continuously as possible, especially at night.

Ribs—Ribs are frequently fractured in accidents. Once braced together for healing, a suitable magnetic field should be placed over this bracing. A 5" x 12" double magnet, multi-magnet flexible mat is usually adequate for treating a cracked rib that is not broken. In the case of a single break, place a 2" x 5" x ¹/₂" magnet over the break or on top of the flexible mat directly over the break. Placing these magnets over the chest will also magnetize the oxygen in the lungs, producing a systemic as well as local treatment.

Joints (Elbows, Knees, Shoulders)—All structures of a joint (bone surfaces, cartilage, and tendons) have to be considered for treatment. In a recent study involving 3,014 patients with joint pain, magnet therapy provided good results in 78.8% of cases.[4] In order to provide continuous treatment, the joint should be wrapped in either a 5" x 6" or 5" x 12" double magnet, multi-magnet flexible mat. Use a 1¹/₂" x ¹/₂" ceramic disc, a 2" x 5" x ¹/₂" ceramic magnet, or a 4" x 6" x ¹/₂" magnet to increase the depth of magnetic field penetration. Although these larger ceramic magnets may not be practical in all cases, they should be used in addition to the flexible mat as often as possible. The magnets can be placed on top of suitable bandages or bracing, which may be required for a joint.

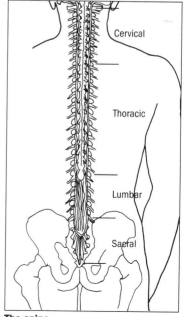

Spine—The spine requires special consideration due to its multiplicity of types of injury to both the vertebrae and the discs between the vertebrae. Ceramic magnets should be used in treating the spine because of their greater depth of penetration. First, place a multi-magnet flexible mat on the injured area. A 5" x 6" double magnet, multi-magnet flexible mat may serve adequately for the cervical spine, but typically use a 5" x 12" double magnet, flexible mat on the lumbar,

The spine.

169

thoracic, or cervical areas of the spine. Wear as many 4" x 6" x $\frac{1}{2}$" magnets as needed up and down the spine for as long as needed. Sleeping on a magnetic bed pad at night is also useful. Sitting on a magnetic chair pad, which has mini-block magnets in the seat cushion as well as up the back, is useful for the lumbar and lower thoracic spine.

Spinal discs have been treated without operation by using a negative magnetic field. Suitable magnets include the 5" x 6" or 5" x 12" double magnet multi-magnet flexible mats. The 4" x 6", 4" x 12", or longer lengths of the plastiform material can also be used. The 4" x 6" x $\frac{1}{2}$" ceramic magnet penetrates more deeply. Sleeping on a negative magnetic field bed pad is helpful. It will take anywhere from six months to a year to heal a disc. If an operation has been performed, then treat the area for several months afterwards; this will aid in healing and help soften up and even remove scar tissue from the surgery.

For more on **headaches**, see *Alternative Medicine Definitive Guide to Headaches* (Future Medicine Publishing, 1997; ISBN 1-887299-18-1); to order, call 800-333-HEAL.

Headaches—Any area of the brain that has been injured has a compromised metabolism due to infections or maladaptive reactions, or other reasons, and can relay pain. Ceramic disc magnets placed bitemporally are usually adequate for treating headaches. They relieve pain by calming the amygdala, which is a center for electrical activity in the brain (located in the temple). Treatment directly over the central cortex (sensory cortex) may also prove to be of value.

Respiratory Problems

FOR THE MILLIONS of people with respiratory difficulties, the simple act of breathing can be a constant struggle. Breathing is almost taken for granted, but has a profound effect on our overall health. The lungs relentlessly pump oxygen which helps rejuvenate blood vessels, digest food, stimulate the heart, and maximize brain function. The lungs also act as a major eliminative organ, where gaseous exchange can be accomplished.

The respiratory system is a complex and sensitive network of organs which provides an immediate link with changes in the atmosphere. There are miles of air passages in the lungs, but by the time air reaches them, it has already been warmed and moistened by the nose, filtered through nose hairs and lymph tissue in the throat, and then constantly refiltered through millions of tiny cilia (hairlike projections along membranous cell tissue) to remove any particles which could damage the lungs.[1]

Respiratory problems can be caused by any number of factors, including viral and bacterial infections, pollen, environmental pollution, and smoking, as well as by a poor quality diet, food toxins and allergies, a stressful and inactive lifestyle, and the misuse of antibiotics. Respiratory problems also manifest in a variety of symptoms related to any one of a number of troublesome conditions. These include hay fever, bronchial asthma, bronchitis, colds and sinusitis, laryngitis, and lung infections.

Asthma

Asthma is the leading cause of disease and disability in children and teens between the ages of two and 17. It is also relatively common among all

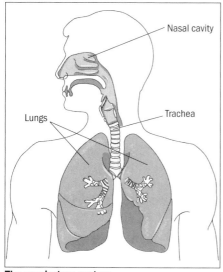
The respiratory system.

age groups, occurring in one out of 40 people, with 65% of sufferers developing symptoms before the age of five.[2] Asthma generally manifests itself in the form of an asthma attack. Between these attacks, an asthmatic will usually seem perfectly healthy. An attack is characterized by a narrowing of the bronchial passages, along with an excessive excretion of mucus, resulting in impaired breathing, with the severity of the symptoms often accelerating rapidly. The greater the obstruction, the more difficult breathing will become.

An attack will usually begin with an unproductive cough, followed by rapidly progressing difficulty in breathing. While the respiratory rate does not increase, expiration becomes prolonged and labored, resulting in wheezing that can often be heard from a distance.[3]

A number of allergic and environmental agents can bring on asthma attacks, including pollen, dust, mold, animal dander, feathers, textiles such as cotton and flax, detergents, petrochemicals, air pollution, and smoke. According to James Braly, M.D., Medical Director of the Immuno Labs in Fort Lauderdale, Florida, wheat, milk, and eggs are among the most likely foods that will trigger an asthma attack. He adds that chemical additives such as food coloring and food preservatives can also be at fault. Sensitivity to aspirin, exposure to cold air, and exercise can also prompt an asthmatic reaction.

Maladaptive reactions to foods, mostly non-immunologic addictions, are a frequent cause of asthma. The cause of asthma cannot be complete until these maladaptive reactions are assessed, using a five-day fast and food testing.

Asthma that originates during infancy is generally due to food allergies; when it strikes between the ages of ten and 30, it is usually due to inhalants; and when it occurs after age 45, it is commonly due to infections. Asthma attacks that occur only in the summer are normally caused by pollens or mold spores, while those that occur only in winter are usually due to infections. And attacks that occur at night tend to be emotionally related and may be due to suppressed anger.

In addition, up to 90% of asthmatics are or were mouth breathers (versus breathing through the nose), making it much easier for dust, pollution, organisms, and cold air to enter the lungs. Breath retraining can be of immense help in alleviating this additional cause of asthma.[4]

Treatment Options for Asthma

The most common medications used by conventional medicine in the treatment of asthma include prednisone, a cortisone derivative, which can cause severe adverse reactions, including fluid and electrolyte disturbances, muscle weakness, peptic ulcers, impaired wound healing, headaches and dizziness, menstrual irregularities, and glaucoma. Prednisone may also help manifest latent diabetes.[5] Approaches such as diet, nutrition, and magnet therapy have shown positive results in the treatment of asthma, without the negative side effects associated with drug-based therapies.

Diet and Nutrition—"Strengthening the immune system is of primary concern in the treatment of asthma," states Dr. Braly. This can be accomplished by eliminating allergens in foods, correcting digestive problems, establishing the proper balance of essential fatty acids, such as those found in cold water fish, and supplying other nutrients important to the immune system.

For the **Four-Day Diversified Rotation Diet**, see Appendix.

In addition, good dietary management needs to be maintained in order to resist asthma. According to Dr. Braly, this can be accomplished by rotating the diet, and avoiding all artificial colorings (especially FD&C Yellow No. 5—tartrazine) and flavorings. He also advises avoiding caffeine, alcohol, tobacco, sugar, and all preservatives.

In addition to eliminating allergic foods, supplementing the diet may help, with nutrients such as vitamins C, B6, B12, and niacinamide, magnesium chloride, and calcium glycerophosphate. For acute asthma attacks, an intravenous injection of these same vitamins and minerals may be required. Other nutrients of direct benefit to asthmatic patients include quercetin (a flavonoid found in onions), beta carotene, selenium, and manganese.

Magnet Therapy—Placing magnets on the front and back of the chest can be a very effective treatment for asthma. However, this treatment may not result in a complete reversal in the most acute phase of asthma. Use either the 5" x 12" double magnet, multi-magnet flexible mat or the 4" x 12" plastiform magnet. The negative magnetic field will relieve the edema and inflammation of the asthma attack, but will not dilate the bronchial tubes. An increased anti-inflammatory value can be achieved by placing the 4" x 6" x ½" magnet over the sternum, which is directly over the bronchi. The asthma attack should eventually subside. Keep in mind, however, that all asthma cases of necessity must be kept under medical supervision.

Bronchitis

Bronchitis refers to a severe inflammation of the bronchial tubes, with symptoms ranging from chills, fever, and coughing, to difficulty breathing and pain in the chest. Acute bronchitis is a mild, short attack, sometimes accompanied by a secondary bacterial infection, while chronic bronchitis is characterized by constant inflammation, often accompanied by irritation of the bronchi, but without any infectious component.

Bronchitis can be caused by infection, exposure to cold, or noxious agents. It is seen much more commonly in the winter as it usually follows some form of upper respiratory infection, such as a cold. In addition, food or chemical allergies can provoke symptoms of bronchitis. Smokers or those exposed to excessive second-hand smoke may also be more vulnerable to chronic bronchitis.

Treatment Options for Bronchitis
In most cases of bronchitis, it is important for mucus to be cleared from the lungs. Coughing can help this, therefore cough suppressants should be avoided unless the patient is extremely weak from lack of sleep. Patients who cough once a minute for 20 minutes have shown a 41% clearance of mucus from the lungs in X rays.[6]

Diet and Nutrition—Dairy products, starches, sugars, and eggs should be avoided in order to produce less mucus. In addition, a whole foods diet will strengthen the immune system, and drinking lots of fresh fluids is essential. Vitamin A has been shown to be effective in relieving bronchitis, as have vitamins C and E. Zinc, proteolytic enzymes (taken between meals), garlic, selenium, and bioflavonoids are other beneficial supplements.

Magnet Therapy—Magnet therapy has been shown effective in treating bronchial inflammation.[7] When treating bronchitis, place either a 5" x 12" double magnet, multi-magnet flexible mat or a 4" x 12" plastiform magnet across the front and back of the chest. Even more importantly, place a 4" x 6" x $1/2$" magnet on top of either or both of these mats, directly over the most affected area. Treatment should last 3-6 hours a day. If possible, the same magnetic therapy should be done throughout the night.

In addition, breathe oxygen (produced by an oxygen concentrator) as much as possible during the bronchitis flare-up. To magnetize oxygen, the tubing goes through a 4" x 6" x 1" ceramic magnet in a wooden frame. Breathing oxygen becomes much more effective for respiratory problems when it is magnetized before it enters the body. The magnets placed directly on the chest also magnetize the oxygen in the lungs and have an additional beneficial effect. Coughing can often be stopped by placing a 4" x 6" x $1/2$" magnet directly over the sternum.

For example, John suffered from chronic bronchitis requiring the constant use of oxygen. When the oxygen was magnetized, John was able to cough up the mucus without the use of medications and able to sleep again with comfort.

Colds and Sinusitis

All of us have experienced the sore throat, runny nose, aching, and general sense of misery that announce the onset of the common cold. Other familiar signals include a cough, headache, and dry, sore, or sensitive breathing passages. In a given year, nearly half of the U.S. population will "catch" a cold and 40% will develop influenza, or the flu.[8]

The symptoms of both the common cold and the flu are often used somewhat interchangeably because both are caused by the same family of respiratory viruses. The distinction between the two depends on how severe the infection is and the range of symptoms. The flu, however, is usually more severe, develops quickly, and involves more of the body than a cold. A cold also occurs at any time of year while the flu, by contrast, usually develops in epidemics, normally in late fall and winter.

The flu produces a moderate to high fever, aching muscles, and acute fatigue. Vomiting and diarrhea may also develop and, in extreme cases, the flu may lead to pneumonia in particularly susceptible individuals. Other complications of the flu, although rare, include inflammation of the brain (encephalitis) or heart (myocarditis), Reye's syndrome (a syndrome primarily affecting children, involving abnormal brain and liver function), and croup.

Sinusitis is an unpleasant and often painful aggravation of the common cold or hay fever, resulting from the inflammation or infection of the air-filled bony cavities that surround the nasal passages. Negative pressure from trapped oxygen can build up inside the sinuses, causing extreme pain. If this swelling remains for any length of time, nature responds by filling the sinus cavity with a thin fluid excreted through the pores of the mucous membrane. This becomes an ideal medium for bacterial growth.

The symptoms of a sinus infection are general malaise, fever, thick discharge from the nose, a nasal voice, and facial pain or headache that is aggravated by bending forward. Only a small percentage of colds progress to sinusitis, however.

With chronic sinusitis, prolonged or repeated inflammation in the nasal passages can lead to degeneration in the tissues that make up the sinus' mucous membrane, hampering the ability of the sinus to drain properly. The main symptoms of this condition are a dull pain over the involved sinus, persistent nasal congestion, thick discharge, chronic postnasal drip, and a diminished sense of smell.

Viruses are commonly thought to be the cause of colds and flu. However, William M. Cargile, B.S., D.C., F.I.A.C.A., counters this belief. "When everyone in the workplace and at home seems to have a cold or the flu, why do some of my patients not get it?" he asks. "I treat people with the flu all day. Why don't I get it?"

Dr. Cargile believes some patients can resist viral attacks, while the immune systems in others are weakened and run down to such a degree that they become susceptible to a viral assault. He says, "It comes down to available energy. The chemicals in the body that regulate stress are deficient and as a result the ability to adapt to stress is diminished. These are the kinds of people who are much more susceptible to getting the flu every year."

Treatment Options for Colds and Sinusitis

"We have between 4,000 and 5,000 microbes of bacteria, viruses, and fungi, living in and on every pore and hole in our bodies," says Dr. Cargile. "The real key to health lies in limiting their populations through dietary control and eating the right foods." Getting extra sleep, cutting simple sugar intake, and drinking large amounts of water, vegetable juices, and broths for a dehydrated respiratory tract, will strengthen immune function and enhance detoxification.

Nutritional Supplements—Many nutritional supplements can be valuable aids in dealing with colds and flu, due to their ability to stimulate immune functions and protect the body from the effects of stress.

The most well-known nutrient for combating colds and flu is vitamin C. Numerous studies have shown that people taking megadoses of vitamin C (amounts far larger than the U.S. RDA standards) report reductions in "the incidence, severity, and duration of colds."[9] After several double-blind studies, researchers found that "vitamin C supplementation may be useful for lessening the severity of disease as well as reducing transmission of viruses."[10] Beyond its antiviral and antibacterial properties, vitamin C acts as an immuno-stimulant. It enhances white blood cell production, increases interferon (a group of proteins released by white blood cells that combat a virus) levels and antibody responses, promotes secretion of thymic hormones, and improves connective tissue.[11]

Garry F. Gordon, M.D., of Payson, Arizona, also recommends zinc throat lozenges, another important nutrient for maintaining the immune system, and thymus extract, which enhances the protective effect of the thymus gland.

Magnet Therapy—If developing a cold, treat the sinuses with a negative magnetic field. Use a magnetic light shield and place a 1" x $\frac{1}{8}$" neodymium disc magnet directly over each sinus. Use at night during sleep. Another method is to tape a 1" x $\frac{1}{2}$" neodymium disc magnet over each infected sinus or over the nose, being careful to always use the negative magnetic field.

Treat the lungs in the front and back with a 5" x 12" double magnet, flexible mat or a 4" x 12" plastiform magnet. Either of these magnets can help prevent the cold from penetrating into the lungs. If the cold is already in the lungs, be sure to treat the lungs in the same manner as mentioned above for bronchitis.

Laryngitis

Laryngitis is inflammation of the larynx. Symptoms include a dry or sore throat, hoarseness, and coughing. To treat laryngitis, place a 5" x 6" double magnet, multi-magnet flexible mat around the neck. Also, place a neodymium or ceramic disc magnet directly over the larynx, held in place with a 2" x 26" band. Maintain this treatment during the night and, when convenient, during the day as well.

Lung Infections

Acute and chronic lung infections, whether viral, bacterial, or fungal, can be treated with a negative magnetic field. First, place a 5" x 12" double magnet, multi-magnet flexible mat or a 4" x 12" plastiform magnet over the front and back of the chest. On top of these mats, place a 4" x 6" x $^{1}/_{2}$" magnet on the mid-sternum, held in place with a 4" x 52" body wrap with shoulder straps or a garment with a pocket to hold this magnet in place. Also, breathe magnetized oxygen as much as possible during the day and night.

Seizures

SEIZURES CAN BE DEFINED as a variety of nonvoluntary contractions (single or in a series) of the voluntary muscles, due to sudden uncontrolled changes in the electrical activity of the brain. Symptoms occur in varying degrees, from mild—with only slight muscle twitches and tingling—to violent, jerking whole-body movements. These are often associated with intense feelings of fear, possible hallucinations, and sometimes a lapse of consciousness. Epileptic seizures with loss of consciousness are called grand mal seizures. While seizures are the major symptom of epilepsy, not all seizures are due to epilepsy.

CAUTION

Seizures can be due to brain tumors or other brain dysfunction. These should be ruled out medically before pursuing alternative treatment.

A seizure disorder is not a disease but a manifestation of underlying brain dysfunction. These brain dysfunctions include perinatal insults, hereditary conditions, trauma, infections, toxic-metabolic disorders, degenerative diseases, tumors, vascular disorders, immunological disturbances, and non-immunologic maladaptive food reactions. A seizure occurs when the brain reaches a high level of electromagnetic excitement. The electroencephalogram and more recently the magnetoencephalogram have made it possible to isolate electromagnetic excitement in the human brain associated with seizure disorders. These instruments have also helped to isolate some focal causes of seizures, such as tumors.

While drug management of seizures is sometimes effective and life-saving, the serious side effects of seizure-control medication, which include growth retardation and reduced learning, offer reasons to pursue the basic causes of seizures and the non-harmful magnetic management for seizure control.

What Causes Seizures?

Some areas of concern for those experiencing seizures, such as tumors, acute toxicities, vascular accidents, and acute encephalitis, are relatively easy to detect during an initial examination. However, other less dramatic and less obvious areas are often neglected, including maladaptive food, chemical, and inhalant reactions as well as nutritional deficiencies. The most neglected area in seizure research is maladaptive food sensitivity reactions, which should be routinely considered in all seizure cases. Maladaptive reactions are the main cause of about 50% of seizures and should constitute a primary part of a comprehensive examination.

There is increasing evidence that free radicals can cause seizures because they irritate the central nervous system. Thus, it is important to use nutritional antioxidants like vitamin C, vitamin E, taurine, glutathione, and selenium in order to reduce any seizure-producing free radicals. Other nutrient deficiencies implicated in seizures include the B vitamins, especially folic acid and vitamin B6, as well as mineral deficiencies including magnesium, calcium, manganese, and zinc.

Fluoride has seizure-inducing effects. It decreases calcium in the blood by combining with it to form an insoluble compound called calcium fluoride. At the same time, the parathyroid glands are extremely sensitive to fluoride. Continuous doses cause hyperparathyroidism, which further decreases calcium, which can result in seizures.[1]

Hypoglycemic episodes—a manifestation of food addictions—can also evoke seizures.

Success Stories: Magnets Relieve Seizures

Henry, 29, was diagnosed with chronic Epstein-Barr viral infection and seizures that produced jerking motions. The seizures and the jerking motion were minimized by placing the negative magnetic field of a 3" x 24" magnet directly on the spine.

After a serious car accident, Brent suffered with grand mal seizures every two hours, day and night. His seizures could not be controlled by any medication. After his seizures, he was like a zombie most of the time. However, his parents decided to use magnetic therapy. After placing $1\frac{1}{2}$" x $\frac{1}{2}$" ceramic disc magnets bitemporally, Brent was seizure-free.

Kevin, 11, had a history of seizures. Several foods, when eaten during a food test, evoked seizures; for example, after eating eggs, he lost motor control of his right hand, widened his eyes as if startled, began drooling, and manifested restless movement of both his arms. These symptoms lasted for 45 seconds and he then slept soundly for two hours. Two weeks later, the same egg test was administered again. This time, however, the negative magnetic field of two ceramic disc magnets were placed bitemporally before the meal and held in place for two more hours. Kevin was completely symptom-free during and after this food test.

Treatment Options for Seizures

Any seizure treatment program should include examining for nutritional deficiencies and genetic errors of metabolism, as well as maladaptive reactions. A Four-Day Diversified Rotation Diet should be implemented at the beginning of the treatment. All potentially addictive substances must be avoided, including tobacco, alcohol, caffeine, and other drugs. Viral infections and toxic states should be treated with intravenous vitamin C, suitable magnetic field exposure, and magnetized oxygen.

In magnetic therapy for seizures, exposing the brain or spine to a positive magnetic field excites the central nervous system. In contrast, exposing the brain or spine to a negative magnetic field is calming. While placing a positive magnetic field directly over a seizure focal area, an electroencephalogram (EEG) shows the seizure pattern, but a negative magnetic field over this same area normalizes the EEG pattern.

A negative magnetic field normalizes the pH of brain cells, shifting them from a diseased acid state to a healthy alkaline state. Also, a negative magnetic field activates the oxidoreductase enzymes, which release oxygen for use by the cells of the brain. By normalizing pH and increasing oxygen to the brain, a negative magnetic field is an anti-inflammatory, anti–free radical, antiviral, antifungal, anti-parasitic, and antibacterial energy force that can significantly reduce all kinds of seizures.

The negative magnetic field should always be placed directly over the foci of central nervous system electrical activity in order to have a calming effect. Otherwise, the symptomatic area can become sufficiently active to evoke a seizure. Trial and error is necessary to discover correct placement and necessary gauss strength for magnetic control of seizures. Suitable magnets include 2" or 3" x $\frac{1}{8}$" plastiform magnets, $1\frac{1}{2}$" x $\frac{1}{2}$" ceramic disc magnets, 1" x $\frac{1}{8}$" neodymium magnets, or 4" x 6" x $\frac{1}{2}$" ceramic magnets. The ceramic magnets have the greatest penetration levels of all these magnets.

Initially use a 24-hour bitemporal exposure until the seizures are completely controlled. Then introduce the Sleep Enhancer at the crown of the head at night; this consists of four 4" x 6" x 1" ceramic magnets placed ³/₄" apart in an adjustable carrier. Be sure the head stays within the magnetic field. If a focus of abnormal electrical activity in the brain is demonstrated with an EEG, then place the magnets over this area.

Nutritional Recommendations

For those experiencing seizures, instead of deliberate food testing, assume that foods eaten twice per week or more, as well as chemicals and inhalants, are potential reactors. Initially, eliminate these foods in a Four-Day Diversified Rotation Diet for three months. At the same time, all potentially damaging chemicals and inhalants must be kept to a minimum.

It is important to supplement with antioxidants such as vitamins C and E, taurine, glutathione, and selenium to reduce any free radicals.

For the **Four-Day Diversified Rotation Diet**, see Appendix.

A double-blind study found that 400 IU of vitamin E daily resulted in six of 12 children having a 90%-100% reduction in seizures. Four of the other children had a 60%-90% reduction in seizures. The last two children had less than a 60% reduction in seizures.

The amino acid taurine is also a great buffer against free radicals. Taurine content is much higher in the central nervous system than in other body tissues. It is necessary for taurine to be in adequate amounts to prevent seizures; cystine is the precursor to taurine. Therefore, cystine and taurine are useful supplements for those having seizures.

To avoid seizures, it is also important to have sufficient B vitamins, especially folic acid and vitamin B6, as well as the minerals magnesium, calcium, manganese, and zinc.

Keep in mind, however, that a negative magnetic field is an excellent free-radical scavenger and can calm the brain and control seizures even in nutritionally deficient people.

Skin Problems

A NUMBER OF CONDITIONS affect the health of the skin, including boils, burns, infections, moles, and warts. Magnet therapy offers real and lasting treatment for skin disorders, without the life-long dependence or side effects of conventional drug therapy.

Boils

A boil is a pus-filled, inflamed area of the skin that can occur anywhere on the body, usually at an infected hair follicle. Most common sites are low back, thighs, buttocks, back of the neck, and armpits. The infection is usually due to the bacteria *Staphylococcus aureus*. A boil usually starts as a painful, slightly red bump, which then becomes more swollen and painful, redder, and filled with pus. It gets a yellowish-white tip and will keep draining or causing pain until the "core," a sac surrounding the pus, is expelled. Recurrent boils may occur in people with decreased immune function, diabetes, chronic gastrointestinal problems, underactive thyroid, or lowered resistance due to nutrient deficiencies and chronic emotional stress.

Treatment Options for Boils

Dietary adjustments that are helpful for boils include eating more green, orange, and yellow vegetables, which are cleansing; try to have at least four different types of green vegetables a day as often as possible, for at least six months. Increase fluids—drink water throughout the day, and drink water with the juice of a fresh lemon and one teaspoon of chlorophyll on rising and before bed. A cleansing fast may be helpful for some people (be sure to build up the immune system after-

For the **Four-Day Diversified Rotation Diet**, see Appendix.

ward). Check for nutritional deficiencies, particularly over-consumption of sugar and white flour products.

Nutrients that may be helpful include: garlic capsules, chlorophyll, pancreatic enzymes (taken on an empty stomach two to three times daily), vitamin E, coenzyme Q10, kelp, zinc, beta carotene, and vitamin A. Emphasize the role of building up the immune system and liver function, and in reducing chronic emotional stress, in the case of chronic boils. Also, consider thymus glandular, one gram of B5 four times daily, vitamin C (one gram every hour), adrenal glandulars, liver-cleansing programs, and bowel-cleansing programs.

The application of a negative magnetic field is an antibiotic and will help reduce the pain and inflammation of boils. For example, Richard had a raised and tender area on his buttocks, which rapidly developed into a boil. It was convenient for him to sit on a 4" x 6" x ½" ceramic magnet for half of the day. After the first two days of this magnetic exposure, the tender area receded. By the third day, the boil was completely gone. Always use a magnet that is larger than the size of the area affected.

Burns

A burn is defined as a heating of the skin (anything over 120° F) so that damage occurs. Symptoms are usually categorized as follows:

■ First degree burns—skin reddens, as only the top layer of the skin is affected (epidermis); skin may peel away in several days and heals quickly.

■ Second degree burns—blisters are created due to damage to the deeper layer of the skin; usually heals without scarring.

■ Third degree burns—the full thickness of the skin is damaged by the heat; area looks charred or white, and tissues below bones and muscles may be exposed; requires burn specialist to treat properly.

Treatment Options for Burns

Superficial burns can be successfully treated with a negative magnetic field that is larger than the burned area. Suitable magnets include the 1½" x ½" ceramic disc or the 1" x ¼" neodymium disc. The plastiform magnetic material can also be cut into any size needed for treating burns. The treatment should occur as quickly as possible after the burn. Relief from pain will usually occur within ten minutes, but it is better to leave the magnet on for 30 minutes or longer; continue treatment until the pain is completely gone.

Usually, blistering will not occur if the magnetic treatment is done immediately. However, if this is not possible, it will still be beneficial to treat the burn in order to prevent infection, increase healing, and prevent scarring. To accomplish this, the magnet should be left on for an extended period of days or even weeks.

For example, Jim burned his finger with steam, an extremely painful type of burn. The finger was immediately packed in ice for ten minutes. After 15 minutes, a blister was already forming. At this point, Jim decided to place his finger on the negative side of a 4" x 6" x ½" ceramic magnet. The blister receded after only 15 minutes and the pain subsided within one hour of magnetic exposure. Two weeks later, the superficial skin peeled, leaving normal new skin.

June scorched the ends of her fingers while testing the burner on an electric stove. Her fingertips quickly turned white and became extremely painful. She immediately placed her fingertips on the negative side of a 300-gauss magnet. Within five minutes, the pain was gone and, after 15 minutes, a normal pink color returned to the scorched area. Blistering and peeling did not occur.

No matter what degree of burn, negative magnetic field therapy can prevent infections and govern healing.

Diet and Nutrition—Consume a high-protein diet for second and third degree burns to promote repair of damaged tissue. Increase your intake of fluids. Eat high-zinc foods such as pumpkin seeds and oysters. Nutrients that may be helpful include: vitamins A, B5 (pantothenic acid), B complex, C (with bioflavonoids) and E, zinc, and free-form amino acids. Spray the burned area with a vitamin C solution. Vitamin E can have a dramatic effect on burns of all kinds: fire, chemical, electrical, and sunburn. Apply 100% solution of dimethylsulfoxide (DMSO) to minimize scarring and prevent loss of skin.

Fever Blisters

For fever blisters, treat the mouth and lips directly with a negative magnetic field that is larger than the blistered area. Suitable magnets include the 1½" x ½" ceramic or the 1" x ⅛" neodymium disc magnets. These magnets should be placed directly on the blistered area at night when asleep as well as whenever convenient during the day. The treatment will take several days to kill the viral infection that usually causes fever blisters.

Insect Stings and Bites

A negative magnetic field exposure effectively stops the inflammation of an insect bite or sting. Insect bites and stings cause an acidic and inflammatory reaction around the affected area. A negative magnetic field quickly changes the acidity of the bite or sting to alkalinity, which often immediately relieves the pain.

If the magnetic treatment is immediate, any inflammation associated with the bite or sting either does not develop or is soon alleviated. The magnet should be left in place until there is no evidence of inflammation. Any size magnet can be used as long as it is larger than the symptomatic area. Typically, the ceramic disc or neodymium disc magnets serve best to relieve all symptoms.

Scalp Infections

Bacterial or fungal infections of the scalp can be treated with a magnetic field. It will take two or more weeks to kill these types of infections. A 5" x 6" double magnet, multi-magnet flexible mat (containing plastiform magnet strips) should be fastened directly on the scalp. It is also possible to use a 4" x 6" plastiform magnet. Cover these magnets with a fabric, such as a washcloth, in order to absorb any perspiration.

Scars

Scars develop due to a lack of oxygen during the healing process. It is important to treat scars, because they continue to send an electromagnetic positive signal of injury to the brain, leading to chronic irritation. Applying a negative magnetic field can cause an initial softening of the tissue and will eventually cause the complete disappearance of a scar after several months of application. Continue the magnetic treatment of the scar tissue as many hours a day as possible, and continue treatment until the scar reverts back to normal skin tissue. If there is a cut on the skin, place a negative magnetic field over this cut, to heal the cut faster and to prevent the formation of any scar. Always use a magnet that is larger than the scar or cut being treated.

Warts and Moles

True warts are very common, contagious skin tumors (benign), "bumps," or "growths," which are caused by at least 35 different viruses. Some warts can turn into cancerous tumors. However, the term *wart* is loosely used for many benign, skin, "wartlike" structures that are not caused by a virus, such as a raised, darkened skin tumor, common in the elderly, called a senile wart or verrucae, that is actually nonviral and more related to aging.

Warts may occur singly or in clusters. Their appearance and size varies tremendously, depending on where they erupt on the body and the degree of irritation or trauma they receive through daily contact. The most common wart (*Verrucae vulgaris*) is a well-defined, rough-surfaced, roundish or irregular growth that may be light gray, brown, grayish-black, or yellow, and is usually firm to the touch. This wart most commonly appears on the knees, elbows, fingers, face, and scalp.

Periungual warts occur around the nail beds. Plantar warts occur on the sole of the foot, are very common, and often appear flattened due to the pressure of walking on them. They are distinguished from other foot growths (corns, calluses) by the fact that, when they are scratched, they "pinpoint" bleed. They may be incredibly painful but this does not necesarily indicate something serious. Warts that appear on a stalk (pedunculated) are common as humans age, particularly around the neck, chest, face, scalp, and armpits. Warts that are common on the face (eyelids, lips, neck) may appear as yellowish long, narrow, small growths.

Warts usually disappear on their own, without any treatment, within several months. However, in some individuals, they may continue for years or reoccur at the same or different parts of the body. Warts in general are more common in older children and usually do not occur in elderly individuals. However, the elderly are prone to other nonviral skin growths such as aging spots.

Mole is a loose term applied to almost any pigmented skin blemish or "growth" that is not viral in origin and may be congenital. They are usually not serious unless irritated constantly or change color, turn darker, or start to bleed.

Treatment Options for Warts and Moles

When warts and moles are exposed to a negative magnetic field, they dry up and peel off, leaving normal skin. Warts generally respond faster than moles; they may require only a few days of exposure to recede; moles may take weeks or months to clear up. For warts or moles that are less than 1" across, the 1" x ⅛" super neodymium disc magnet is ideal for treatment. If the lesion is larger than one inch, then the 1½" x ½" ceramic disc magnet is the magnet of choice. Hypoallergenic tape (such as HY tape) can be used to hold magnets in place. For raised and sore lesions, place a corn cushion pad around the lesion, then place the magnet on top of the pad.

Several nutrients are helpful for treating warts and moles: vitamin A (100,000 IU for five days, then reduce to 25,000 IU for one month); beta carotene (50,000 IU for several weeks); vitamin C; L-cysteine (500 mg two times daily for one month, with an amino acid blend one time daily); vitamin B complex; zinc; and vitamin E.

Sunburn

Sunburn is an overexposure of the skin to ultraviolet radiation (sunlight), leading to inflammation and burns of the skin. This occurs more frequently in fair-skinned individuals. Symptoms appear up to 24 hours after exposure and peak at 72 hours, unless the burning is severe. The affected skin turns anywhere from mildly reddish to severely red and darker. Symptoms range from skin becoming mildly tender to severe pain and swelling. Blisters may appear, which then open and the outer layer of the skin peels away. Sunburn on the lower extremities is usually more painful and takes longer to heal. If a large enough portion of the skin is affected, systemic symptoms may occur, such as chills, fever, weakness, and shock. Secondary infections may follow once the skin has peeled. The new skin may be very sensitive to touch and to further sunlight for several weeks.

Treatment Options for Sunburn

The best treatment is prevention. Initial summer exposure should not exceed 30 minutes during the midday sun, even in persons with darker skin. The best time for sun exposure is before 11 a.m. and after 3 p.m. Cloudy summer days and foggy winter days, especially at higher altitudes, pose a greater danger of sunburn, as they appear to be safer but have almost the same amount of ultraviolet exposure. Reflections off of water, metal, snow, sand, and silvery objects may increase the amount of rays absorbed. Repeated overexposure to the sun and sunburns leads to aging of the skin and increases the risk of skin cancers.

A 5" x 12" double magnet, multi-magnet flexible mat should be placed over any area of the body that has been sunburned. On the outside of the mat, place one or two 1½" x ½" ceramic disc magnets or 1" x ⅛" neodymium disc magnets directly over the sunburned area. These additional magnets will reinforce the depth of the magnetic field. When lying down, place a 4" x 6" x ½" ceramic magnet over the sunburned area.

Nutrients—A number of nutrients can effectively relieve a case of sunburn: vitamin E (orally and topically); vitamin A (for a mild burn—50,000 IU daily for several days; for more severe burns—100,000 IU for first three days, then reduce to 50,000 IU daily for several weeks); vitamin C (amounts of the antioxidants depend on degree of severity); potassium (100 mg once daily for one to two weeks); calcium and magnesium. Also, you can mix together vitamins A and E, essential fatty acids, zinc oxide, and aloe gel, and place on skin.

Sleep Disorders

OVER 50 MILLION Americans suffer from sleep disorders, including insomnia, excessive drowsiness, and restless movement during sleep. According to many practitioners, these disorders often are related to nutritional or behavioral factors, and may be remedied by addressing the various causes and symptoms underlying the condition. Sleep is a restorative process that serves to replenish both physiologically and psychologically. As an essential part of the daily human cycle, sleep is a determining factor in the state of a person's health.

"The quantity and quality of sleep vary from person to person, but how well and how long one sleeps is ultimately the result of varying physical and psychological influences," says John Zimmerman, Ph.D., Laboratory Director of the Washoe Sleep Disorders Center in Reno, Nevada. Not only can stress, illness, and anxiety contribute to sleep disorders, but so can external circumstances such as a noisy sleeping room, as well as disturbed biological rhythms such as those occurring due to night-shift work and jet lag, adds Dr. Zimmerman. A shortened attention span, the loss of physical strength, and difficulty in responding to unfamiliar situations are all common symptoms of sleep disorders.

The Five Stages of Sleep

The first four stages are called NREM (non–rapid eye movement) sleep; the fifth stage is REM (rapid eye movement). The NREM phases comprise approximately 75% of the sleep cycle (50% in infants) and are characterized by very restful sleep, in which body movements, blood pressure, breathing, and basal metabolic rates are reduced by as much as 30% from normal wakeful levels.[1] There may be some dreaming during NREM sleep though you're unlikely to recall them.[2] The majority of remembered dreaming occurs during the REM phase.

In everyone except for infants, narcoleptics, and people deprived of sleep for more than 200 hours, NREM stages precede REM. However, you may skip around from various light and deep stages or completely omit the deep sleep stages after the second or third cycle of the night. Additionally, people commonly experience a period of up to two hours of "quiet wakefulness" between four-hour periods of regular sleep cycles. During this interval, according to studies, sleepers are neither fully awake nor fully asleep, but resting, reviewing their dreams, their thoughts turned off.

Stage 1—This is the shortest phase, in which slowing alpha waves prepare you for the sleep state. As you drift in and out of wakefulness, your breathing, heart rate, metabolic rate, and body temperature begin to drop. Muscles start to relax; you may experience a sensation of falling followed by sudden muscle contractions called hypnic myoclonia. You may experience hypnagogic (the act of falling asleep) dreams. You are easily awakened by external stimuli, at which point you may only remember a few fragments of hypnagogic images and thoughts.

Stage 2—This is the longest sleep phase, marked by a light level of sleep. The brain slows down into theta waves, with intermittent surges of rapid brain waves (spindles) followed by large, slow bursts of delta waves. Breathing, heart rate, metabolic rate, and body temperature continue to decline. You may be awakened easily by sound and movement.

Stage 3—As the brain progressively slows down to large, slow delta waves, you enter a deeper stage of sleep. Muscles go limp and breathing is slow and even. The sleeper may begin to sweat. During this stage and Stage 4, the body begins to restore itself. In people under 30, the endocrine glands release human growth hormone (HGH), which promotes cell division and organ growth.

Awakening a person in Stage 3 sleep is fairly difficult to do, and the sleeper may experience grogginess for a few seconds or minutes after awakening. After two or three sleep cycles, this stage may disappear and you may go directly from Stage 2 to REM sleep.

Stage 4—This is the deepest stage of sleep. Delta waves become larger and much slower than in Stage 3, and breathing, heart rate, metabolism, and temperature reach their lowest levels. Muscles continue to be inactive and the sleeper may sweat, but the body continues its restorative activities. Some sleepers may experience night terrors or sleepwalking. Toward the end of this stage, sleepers may readjust their position and may experience a muscular contraction as they enter the next stage. Rousing sleepers from this phase takes a great deal of effort. Once awakened, people feel groggy and may require several minutes to orient themselves. After two or three cycles, this stage may disappear for the duration of the night.

Stage 5 (REM)—This is the dreaming phase, marked by small, rapid alpha waves that resemble those indicating wakefulness and sensory awareness of external stimuli. However, in this stage our brains are reacting to internally generated stimuli from our dreams. All other muscles seize up to prevent us from reacting to the action in the dreams, but the sleeper may experience some slight twitching in the face, fingers, and toes. Men experience penile erections. Breathing and heart rate speed up and slow down in reaction to dream content. A sleeper in the REM stage is difficult to rouse and, if awakened, they will have a hard time adjusting to reality. This stage becomes progressively longer with each cycle, possibly lasting 60 minutes in the fifth cycle.

Types of Sleep Disorders

Sleep disorders are a particularly troublesome health concern. Not only can they be the result of other, often undetected ailments, but they also generate their own health complications. Insomnia, sleep apnea, and periodic leg movement syndrome (PLMS)/restless leg syndrome are common sleep disorders.

■ Insomnia—Insomnia, characterized by an inability either to fall asleep or to remain asleep during the course of the night, can be traced to a number of physical, mental, behavioral, and situational factors. Insomnia has been classified in terms of the time of night that it effects. There are three main types of insomnia: sleep-onset insomnia, sleep-maintenance insomnia, and early-morning-awakening insomnia. People who take hours to fall asleep but sleep relatively well throughout the remainder of the night have sleep-onset insomnia. Those who wake up several times in the middle of the night and have trouble falling back to sleep suffer from sleep-maintenance insomnia. Individuals who awaken too early have a condition called early-morn-

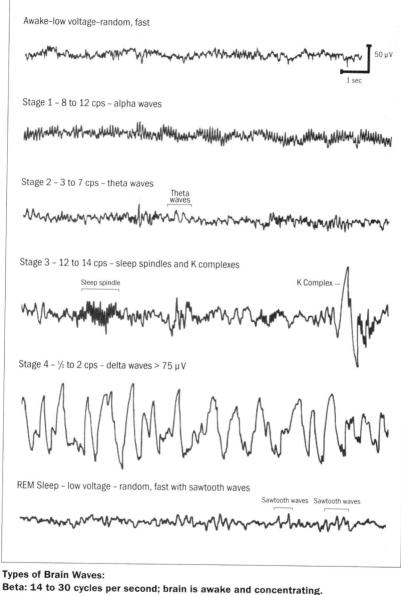

Awake–low voltage–random, fast

50 µV

1 sec

Stage 1 – 8 to 12 cps – alpha waves

Stage 2 – 3 to 7 cps – theta waves

Theta waves

Stage 3 – 12 to 14 cps – sleep spindles and K complexes

Sleep spindle

K Complex —

Stage 4 – ½ to 2 cps – delta waves > 75 µV

REM Sleep – low voltage – random, fast with sawtooth waves

Sawtooth waves Sawtooth waves

Types of Brain Waves:
Beta: 14 to 30 cycles per second; brain is awake and concentrating.
Alpha: 8 to 13 cycles per second; brain is awake but relaxed.
Theta: 4 to 7 cycles per second; brain is sleeping lightly.
Delta: 1 to 3 cycles per second; brain is sleeping deeply with no dreams.

ing-awakening insomnia. Psychophysiological insomnia is an official diagnostic category the symptoms of which often include sleep-onset insomnia. In psychophysiological insomnia, a person's normal presleep rituals, behavior, or sleeping environment trigger insomnia. In this case, the more the sufferer worries about falling asleep, the worse it becomes.

■ Sleep Apnea—Sleep apnea refers to a serious condition in which there is intermittent cessation of breathing during sleep which forces the individual to repeatedly wake up to take breaths of air. This disturbs the continuity of sleep and is a primary cause of the excessive daytime sleepiness associated with this disorder. There are three types of sleep apnea: central sleep apnea, obstructive sleep apnea, and a combination of the first two types called mixed-type sleep apnea. Central sleep apnea refers to a defect in the central nervous system which affects the diaphragm. It can result in poor quality sleep, frequent awakening during the night, and excessive fatigue throughout the day. Obstructive sleep apnea occurs when a blockage develops in the upper airway, preventing normal air flow. Individuals who have obstructive sleep apnea usually snore and are often excessively tired and sleepy throughout the day.

■ Periodic Leg Movements Syndrome and Restless Legs Syndrome—Periodic leg movement syndrome (PLMS) causes repeated leg movements during the onset of sleep or during sleep itself. These occur as a series of stereotyped, repetitive movements throughout the night. A related disorder called restless legs syndrome is characterized by periodic leg movements and uncomfortable leg sensations.

What Causes Sleep Disorders?

Sleep disorders occur for many reasons: psychological (such as anxiety), or biochemical (such as the inappropriate use of sleeping pills or other drugs), or medical (such as the physiological problems often associated with sleep apnea or restless legs syndrome), as well as lifestyle choices (such as poor diet and lack of exercise).

Diet
Diet is a primary factor when considering sleep disorders. Intolerance to certain foods, eating excessively, the consumption of caffeine are important concerns.

■ Caffeine—Caffeine can have a pronounced effect on sleeping habits. Caffeine consumption has been associated with insomnia, periodic leg movements syndrome, and restless legs syndrome. Many over-the-counter medications such as cold and cough preparations that contain caffeine, or caffeine-related substances, can also increase sleep disorders.

■ Food Intolerance—Herbert Rinkel, M.D., former Associate Instructor in Medicine at the University of Oklahoma School of Medicine, is considered one of the first to bring to light the issue of food sensitivities. While still a medical student, he discovered his own intolerance to eggs, and began to research the field. Dr. Rinkel found that symptoms of tension and jitteriness, common to food-sensitive individuals, are apt to manifest in restlessness and inattentiveness by day, and insomnia by night. He concluded that insomnia, as well as tossing about or crying out at night, are very frequent manifestations of food intolerance.

Fatigue is often one of the first symptoms of food intolerance, and is most troublesome early in the morning upon rising. This is particularly noticeable in children with food intolerances. People suffering from food intolerances are often irritable during the morning hours and may need a nap in the late afternoon. They frequently suffer from insomnia as well, according to Dr. Rinkel.[3]

Intolerance to certain foods can cause histamine (a substance produced by the body during an allergic reaction) to be released in the brain, which can disturb a person's biochemistry, and can, in some cases, lead to sleep disturbance. In the brain, histamine replaces neurotransmitters (SEE QUICK DEFINITION), but because it does not function like other neurotransmitters, it creates a dysfunction in the biochemical pathways of the brain (which are responsible for thinking, mood, and behavior). When these pathways are disrupted, the consequence is exhibited as symptoms, one of which is insomnia.

Environmental Factors
"Items that interfere with the body's electromagnetic field and create electromagnetic fields of

QUICK
DEFINITION

A **neurotransmitter** is a brain chemical with the specific function of enabling communications between brain cells, called neurons. Electrical thought impulses are changed into neurotransmitters at the dendrites, the branching tips of a nerve cell; then they are passed on to the next nerve cell. Chief among the 100 neurotransmitters identified to date, there are six involved in most mental activities. These are acetylcholine, gamma-aminobutyric acid (GABA), serotonin, dopamine, L-glutamate, and norepinephrine. *Acetylcholine* is required for short-term memory, concentration, and all muscle contractions. *GABA* is a calming agent that works to stop excess nerve signals (stimulation) and thus keeps brain firings from getting out of control. *Serotonin* does the same and helps produce sleep, regulate pain, and influence mood—it's called the "feel good" neurotransmitter—although too much serotonin can produce depression. *Dopamine* regulates physical movements and muscular control, and it influences mood, sex drive, and memory retrieval. *L-glutamate* is essential for laying down new memories and the recall of existing ones; it also inhibits the chronic stress response and the excess secretion of cortisol. *Norepinephrine* causes the brain to be more alert; it helps carry memories from short-term "storage" to long-term and it enables one to maintain a positive mood.

Circadian Biological Rhythms and Magnetic Fields

Circadian rhythms are regularly recurring, biological changes in our mental and physical behaviors over the course of the day. As indicated by the term *circadian* (Latin for "around a day"), these rhythms repeat approximately every 24 hours and are primarily controlled by the body's biological "clock." Circadian rhythms are most commonly linked to sleep/wake patterns and account for the fluctuations of alertness and drowsiness throughout the day. People with normal circadian rhythms are most alert during the morning and afternoon, but tend to get drowsy toward evening and feel the need for sleep at nighttime.

Research shows that circadian rhythms occur in other physiological processes as well, including blood pressure, body temperature, hormone levels, and the immune system.[4] Light, from both the sun and artificial devices, as well as environmental cues such as alarm clocks, influence our circadian rhythms and set our body clocks to follow the 24-hour cycle of the sun.

The pineal gland secretes melatonin in extremely minute amounts—blood levels of melatonin are measured in *picograms*, that is, trillionths of a gram. The actual amounts depend on age and other factors, but between five and ten times more melatonin is released at night than during the day.[5] Melatonin is the antithesis of another hormone, adrenaline, produced by the adrenal glands. As melatonin enters the bloodstream, it begins to slow down the waking (alpha) brain waves. Subsequently the heart rate decreases, muscles relax, blood pressure drops, and the body begins to enter the stages of sleep.

Many people with sleep disorders have disrupted circadian rhythms, often due to melatonin imbalances, in which the natural sleep–wake patterns are interrupted or reversed. Many Americans

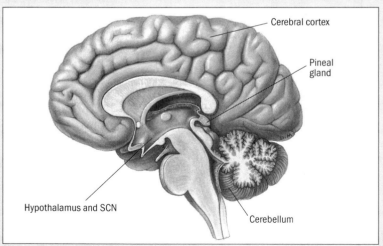

Cerebral cortex

Pineal gland

Hypothalamus and SCN

Cerebellum

Parts of the brain involved in the body clock.

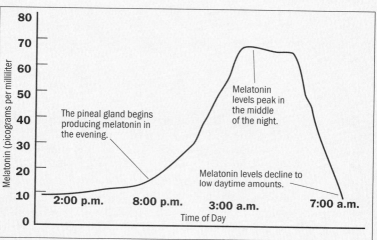

The 24-Hour Cycle of Melatonin Production.

Chart labels:
- Melatonin (picograms per milliliter) — y-axis: 0, 10, 20, 30, 40, 50, 60, 70, 80
- Time of Day — x-axis: 2:00 p.m., 8:00 p.m., 3:00 a.m., 7:00 a.m.
- The pineal gland begins producing melatonin in the evening.
- Melatonin levels peak in the middle of the night.
- Melatonin levels decline to low daytime amounts.

spend up to 90% of their days indoors, in buildings with fluorescent lights. This lack of exposure to bright sunlight or its artificial cousin, full-spectrum light, is a major contributor to disrupted circadian rhythms and concurrent reduced melatonin levels. Lack of regular exercise, structural imbalances, and chronic stress are also common factors. So, too, is a poor diet, often marked by overconsumption of stimulants such as alcohol, coffee, spicy foods, sugar, and over-the-counter medications. Electromagnetic fields, both natural and artificial, also play a role in diminishing the function of the pineal gland, resulting in decreased melatonin production and an imbalanced body clock.

The daytime hours are governed by a positive magnetic field, while the dark is governed by a negative field. The pineal gland, which is a magnetic organ, is sensitive to these daily cyclic shifts of magnetic field. If these daily shifts are altered, and one is exposed to a high positive magnetic field, then the production of melatonin is also altered. A host of symptoms may begin to appear if the conditions become chronic. Your sleep cycles get disrupted and the quantity and quality of your sleep usually suffers.

Rest, relaxation, and especially deep sleep are necessary for recovery of energy expended during the wakeful periods. Negative magnetic field energy can help you keep pace with these changes in circadian rhythm. If you cannot naturally acquire sufficient negative magnetic energy, you must supply it from an external source by applying negative pole magnets to your body.

their own can disrupt sleep," states Anthony Scott-Morley, D.S.C., Ph.D., M.D. (alt. med.), B.A., from Dorset, England. "These include electric blankets, electrically heated waterbeds, electric clocks (at the head of the bed), and 60-cycle frequencies (household electric current), as well as power lines and generators. Also, sleeping near or over geopathic stress zones (areas of harmful Earth radiation) seriously affect the sleep habits of sensitive individuals." Sleep problems can sometimes be attributed to factors like ventilation, humidity, noise, or an uncomfortable mattress.

Treatment Options for Sleep Disorders

The negative magnetic field can influence many biochemical processes within the body that directly relate to maintaining proper sleep patterns. For example, the negative magnetic field is one factor that directly influences the body's acid-alkaline (pH) balance. Oxygen levels are compromised when maladaptive reactions change the cellular and tissue pH in the body to acid. Once oxygen levels are reduced, the painful discomforts of swollen cells may disturb proper sleep patterns. In order to reverse these conditions to the more favorable alkaline and oxygenated conditions necessary for sound sleep, it is important to treat any area of local edema, as well as the entire system, with a negative magnetic field.

Magnetic field therapy is quite effective in treating and preventing all types of sleep disorders. The following are general guidelines that will improve your sleep:

Sleep on a magnetic bed pad composed of mini-block magnets placed sufficiently close together to provide a full negative magnetic field. Exposure to this magnetic bed serves to increase melatonin production, particularly from the intestinal tract wall. The intestinal tract can be further stimulated to make more melatonin by sleeping with a 5" x 12" double magnet, multi-magnet flexible mat held across the abdomen, held in place with a 4" x 52" body wrap.

Sleep with your head in a negative magnetic field—this is even more effective in producing sound sleep than a magnetic bed pad. Place four 4" x 6" x 1" magnets $3/4$" apart in a carrier, which holds them firmly against the headboard. These magnets can be raised or lowered depending on the height of the pillow. The top of the head should be as close as possible to the magnets.

Recently, researchers have generated a great deal of scientific information about the hormone melatonin.[6] Several current books have focused on the value of supplementary melatonin in reversing insomnia as well as preventing and reversing aging. There is a logical concern that supplementary melatonin may suppress some amounts of the normal production of hormones made by the pineal gland. Given the potential problems associated with supplementary melatonin, how can the body be stimulated to produce the hormone naturally? A negative magnetic field actually stimulates the pineal gland, the retina of the eyes, and the intestinal tract wall to produce melatonin. Researchers found measurable evidence of significantly increased electrical activity of the pineal gland when it was exposed to a negative magnetic field.[7] Robert O. Becker, M.D., observed that melatonin secretion may be changed by exposure to a static magnetic field.[8]

For more on **sleep disorders**, see *Sleep Disorders: An Alternative Medicine Definitive Guide* (AlternativeMedicine.com Books, 2000; ISBN 1-887299-20-3); to order, call 800-333-HEAL.

One can achieve the benefits of increased melatonin by sleeping on a negative magnetic field mattress pad, by placing a negative field flexible magnetic pad across the abdomen, by placing a negative magnetic eye unit across the eyes, and, especially, by treating the brain with a negative magnetic field. This treatment method produces energy-restoring deep sleep and all the healing benefits of melatonin.

Since light stops melatonin production, you should sleep in total darkness. The response of the eyes to light cuts off the production of melatonin and growth hormone during sleep. Therefore, if light comes through a window or you sleep in the daytime, wear a pad or light shield over the eyes. Use the magnetic eye unit, composed of a light shield with 1" x $\frac{1}{8}$" neodymium disc magnets over the eyes.

An alternative to the light shield arrangement is to wear a 5" x 12" double magnet, multi-magnet flexible mat over the eyes, placed across the face so both the front and sides of each eye are treated. In addition, place a superneodymium magnet on top of this mat, directly over the side of each eye. Use a 2" x 26" self-fastening band to hold this arrangement in place.

To further stimulate the gastrointestinal tract to produce melatonin, sleep with a 5" x 12" double magnet, multi-magnet flexible pad across the abdomen. Centered over this multi-magnet pad, place a 4" x 6" x $\frac{1}{2}$" ceramic magnet lengthwise on the body. Another method is to use the 4" x 12" x $\frac{1}{8}$" plastiform strips at night while asleep.

Sleep in an environment that has no electric clocks, electric blankets, or 60-cycle electric fields of any kind, which block melatonin production by the pineal gland.

Success Story: Sleep Apnea

Henry, a man in his seventies, experienced sleep apnea, or intermittent cessation of breathing during sleep. This intermittent breathing obviously disturbed his continuity of sleep. Henry corrected this problem in about one year by sleeping with a negative magnetic field at the crown of his head. Consequently, he slept deeper and experienced more energy during the day.

Success Story: Environmental Sleep Problems

Bonnie reported that she could not sleep if the top of her head was near one wall in her bedroom. However, she would sleep well on the opposite side of the room. A magnetometer examination of the room revealed that the wall where she could not sleep registered a positive magnetic field and the wall where she was able to sleep registered a negative magnetic field. The building had an iron framework and the electric currents running through the walls had caused the iron framing to become magnetized, thus setting up opposite magnetic poles. Through understanding the environmental factors disturbing her sleep and making appropriate changes—in this case, simply moving her bed—Bonnie was once again able to get a good night's sleep.

Dietary Changes

Diet is especially important when treating sleep disorders, and it is essential to rule out food intolerances as a cause. In one study of infants, sleeplessness was eliminated by removing cow's milk from the diet and then reproduced by its reintroduction.[9] A combination of nutritional adjustments can also aid sleep, including:

■ No alcohol consumption

■ Avoiding caffeine in all forms (tea, coffee, cola, chocolate)

■ Taking one gram of niacinamide (vitamin B3) at bedtime (for the type that sleeps easily but wakes and cannot get back to sleep)

As much as possible, one should strictly avoid chemicals that reduce melatonin, including caffeine, tobacco, alcohol, beta blockers, calcium channel blockers, sleeping pills, tranquilizers, Prozac, and such nonsteroidal, anti-inflammatory drugs as aspirin, indomethacin, and all common pain-killers.

For food intolerances, use the Four-Day Diversified Rotation Diet and strictly limit the amount of refined sugar intake in the daily diet.

Vitamins

■ The B vitamins are known to have a sedative effect on the nerves, and vitamin B6 supplements can help to prevent insomnia. Vitamin B6 (pyroxidine) strongly influences the immune and nervous systems. Vitamin B6 is needed by the body for the conversion of the amino acid tryptophan to the brain neurotransmitter serotonin, which helps to control sleep. Deficiencies occur as a result of eating a diet high in fats and low in fruits and vegetables.

Food sources: brewer's yeast, whole grains, legumes, nuts, and seeds. Supplements: there are two forms of B6, pyridoxine hydrochloride and pyridoxal-5-phosphate (the most active form). For efficient absorption of pyridoxal by the body, sufficient levels of riboflavin and magnesium should be present.[10] Typical recommended dose: 50-100 mg daily can help to prevent insomnia. Precautions: High levels of pyridoxine can cause toxic side effects.[11]

■ Vitamin B12 is another important supplement to consider when treating insomnia (25 mg of vitamin B12 can serve as an effective anti-insomnia vitamin regimen). The best food sources of the B vitamins are liver, whole grains, wheat germ, tuna, walnuts, peanuts, bananas, sunflower seeds, and blackstrap molasses.

For the **Four-Day Diversified Rotation Diet**, see Appendix.

■ Vitamin E (Alpha Tocopherol)—Vitamin E has been shown effective in treating restless legs syndrome, which may be caused by decreased circulation to the legs. In one study concerning vitamin E and restless legs syndrome, a 78-year-old female with a history of restless and "jumpy" legs found that after two months of 300 IU daily, she was completely cured.[12] In another study, a 37-year-old female with a ten-year history of severe nightly "restless legs" was placed on 300 IU daily for six weeks and 200 IU daily for the following four weeks with complete relief.[13]

Food sources: cold-pressed polyunsaturated vegetable oils (such as sunflower and safflower), leafy green vegetables, avocados, nuts, seeds, and whole grains. Supplements: Vitamin E is actually a group of compounds called tocopherols. When purchasing supplements of vitamin E, avoid products that contain vitamin E in the DL-alpha tocopherol acetate form—this means that it is a petroleum-based synthetic form of the vitamin. The natural form of vitamin E will be designated with the letter "D". Typical recommended dose: 30 IU daily; for those suffering from restless legs syndrome, 800-1,200 IU of vitamin E should be taken per day.

Minerals

■ Calcium—Calcium and magnesium nourish the nervous system and act as natural relaxants. Many people have systems that are too acidic and need to be more alkaline and they benefit from taking these mineral supplements, which are both alkaline and a sedative. Low levels of calcium and magnesium have been associated with muscle cramping, which can disrupt sleep.[14] Calcium absorption into the cells can be compromised by whole grains and cereals, spinach, and by tannins in tea, a diet high in protein, commercial soda, refined sugar, and antacids that contain aluminum.[15]

Food sources: broccoli, cabbage, almonds, hazelnuts, oats, lentils, beans, figs, currants and raisins, Brussels sprouts, cauliflower, kelp, and green leafy vegetables especially kale. Kale is very high in an easily absorbed form of calcium.[16] Supplements: bone meal, dolomite, and oyster shell calcium have been found to have the highest levels of lead and should not be used as a supplement.[17] Calcium citrate and calcium gluconate have a much better absorption level.[18] One of the best forms of absorbable calcium is microcrystalline hydroxyapatite. Typical dose: 600 mg of liquid calcium can have a relaxing effect (take calcium in a 2-to-1 ratio to magnesium). Precautions: Excessive intake of calcium oxalate may cause the formation of kidneys stones, but this risk can be decreased by using the calcium citrate and calcium gluconate forms. High calcium intake can interfere with iron absorption, cause chronic constipation, and may also increase blood pressure.[19]

■ Magnesium—Magnesium is second only to potassium as the most concentrated mineral within the cells. Magnesium helps form bones, relax muscle spasms, and decrease the pain involved in arthritis. It activates cellular enzymes and plays a large role in nerve and muscle function as well as helping to regulate the acid-alkaline balance.[20] Magnesium deficiency can cause anxiety, muscle tremors, confusion, irritability, and pain. Processed food or foods cooked at high temperatures can be depleted of their magnesium content.

Food sources: tofu, nuts and seeds, and green leafy vegetables, especially kale, seaweed and chlorophyll. Supplements: magnesium is absorbed well when taken as an oral supplement and will increase the measurable levels inside red and white blood cells.[21] Use magnesium glycinate, fumerate, or citrate, which are usually better absorbed with less of a laxative effect.[22] Epsom salts (magnesium sulfate), an old-fashioned remedy, is an excellent addition to a bath, but has a strong laxative effect if taken as an oral supplement. Typical dose: 250 mg. Precautions: Very high doses of magnesium may be dangerous if kidney disease is present.

■ Chromium—Chromium is a mineral essential for regulating the production of the hormone insulin, which is responsible for stabilizing blood sugar levels. Although the body requires only small amounts of this important mineral, Americans are more likely to be deficient in chromium than any other micronutrient. Chromium is found in the outer bran portion of grains, but much of it is lost in the milling and processing of white flour (the staple ingredient in most refined bread and pasta products). The chromium that we do draw from food sources can be depleted in our bodies by various means, including a high-carbohydrate diet, infections, and physical and emotional stress.

The urinary excretion of chromium can increase as much as 50-fold under stress.[23] A high intake of white sugar also tends to deplete the body of chromium, as the mineral is used up in removing these sugars from the blood.[24]

Food sources: an excellent source of chromium is brewer's yeast (available in powder form or in tablets), wheat germ, beef and chicken, liver, whole grains, potatoes, eggs, apples, bananas, and spinach. Supplements: Chromium and other minerals are better absorbed in the body when bound in a "transporter" molecule, called a chelate. Chelated minerals are better protected from damage in the digestive system. Glucose tolerance factor chelate (GTF chromium) tends to be a more bioavailable form of chromium than chromium salts, such as chromium chloride.[25] Chromium polynicotinate is another chelated variety that is chemically bound to niacin, a B-complex vitamin. According to some researchers, this form of chromium is superior to either chromium chloride or chromium picolinate. Typical recommended dosage: 250-500 mcg twice a day.

Amino Acids

Amino acids are the building blocks of proteins; in fact, proteins are actually chains of amino acids linked together, each one having a specific function. Proteins are, in turn, the building blocks of the body. Twenty-two amino acids are vital to the body's growth, development, and maintenance. Some are manufactured in the body while others, called essential amino acids, must be obtained from the diet or nutritional supplements. Semi-essential amino acids can be made by the body in amounts that are adequate to maintain basic protein requirements, however, additional dietary sources are required during times of growth or stress. Amino acid deficiency may be an underlying factor, often undetected, for sleep disorders. Vegetarians and vegans (vegetarians who eat no dairy products) often have difficulty meeting dietary protein requirements, and should take an amino acid complex supplement.

■ Tryptophan and 5-HTP—L-tryptophan is considered the best amino acid for sleeping problems. L-tryptophan is a precursor to serotonin, which is then converted into melatonin. The presence of melatonin allows the body to drop off into slumber. Tryptophan occurs naturally in certain foods, including turkey and other meats, milk and cheese, and legumes. Other tryptophan-containing foods include cashews, spinach, bananas, figs, dates, yogurt, tuna, and whole grain crackers. Research shows that tryptophan helps about half of all

For information on
5-HTP, contact:
NutriCology, 400
Preda Street, San
Leandro, CA
94577; tel: 800-
545-9960 or 510-
639-4572; fax:
510-635-6730. Life
Enhancement
Products, Inc., P.O.
Box 751390,
Petaluma, CA
94975; tel: 800-
543-3873 or 707-
762-6144; fax:
707-769-8016.
BioSynergy Health
Alternatives, 106
N. 6th Street, Suite
200, Boise, ID
83702; tel: 800-
554-7145; fax:
208-342-0880.

See *The
Supplement
Shopper* (Future
Medicine
Publishing, 1999;
ISBN 1-887299-17-
3); to order, call
800-333-HEAL.

insomnia sufferers.[26] Unfortunately, L-tryptophan supplements are no longer readily available. During the 1980s, L-tryptophan was sold as a natural, non-habit-forming sleeping aid, until a "bad batch" manufactured in Japan caused more than a thousand people to become ill; it was subsequently banned by the U.S. Food and Drug Administration.

There is, however, a substitute called 5-HTP, or 5-hydoxytryptophan, which is a form of tryptophan that is a step closer to serotonin. Tryptophan is usually converted in the brain into 5-HTP, which is then turned into serotonin. It has been shown to be effective in treating depression, fibromyalgia, headaches, and insomnia.[27] A Norwegian study showed that 5-HTP had an effect on sleep patterns by increasing the levels of serotonin. The researchers injected cats with 5-HTP (40 mg/kg body weight) or L-tryptophan and found that both substances had a "general deactivating effect on the waking state" and produced a deep sleeping state.[28]

The typical recommended dosage of 5-HTP for improving the symptoms of "serotonin deficiency syndrome" is 25-50 mg daily. Higher dosages (over 100 mg) could cause some side effects, including mild nausea. Vitamin B6 should also be taken on the same day as 5-HTP, because it is necessary for converting 5-HTP into serotonin.

■ Phosphatidylserine, an amino acid which helps the hypothalamus regulate the amount of cortisone produced by the adrenals, is helpful for those who cannot sleep because of high cortisone levels, usually induced by stress. Cortisone is usually at high levels in the morning, for wakefulness, but in stressed individuals it may be high at night and prevent sleeping.

Supplements: The preferred amino acid supplements are labeled *USP pharmaceutical grade*, L-crystalline, free-form amino acids. The term *USP* means that the product meets the standards of purity and potency set by the United States Pharmacopeia. The term *free-form* refers to the highest level of purity of the amino acid. The *L* refers to one of the two forms in which most amino acids come, designated D- and L- (as in D-lysine or L-lysine). The L-form amino acids are proper for human biochemistry, as proteins in the human body are made from this form.

Generally, it is not recommended for people to take individual amino acids for extended or indefinite periods as this can create an imbalance of other amino acids in the body and possibly cause other health conditions. If individual amino acids are going to be used to support specific health conditions, follow this course of treatment with a complex of free-form amino acids to ensure balanced amino acid nutrition. Please consult a qualified health-care professional before beginning such therapies. Individual amino acids often come with warnings or precautions for women who are pregnant or for people with certain health conditions.

Women's Health Problems

W O M E N ' S   H E A L T H   C A R E focuses on maintaining optimal health as her reproductive system develops and matures. Conventional approaches to women's health have often used invasive medical procedures to deal with common physiological functions, such as the hormonal imbalances experienced during menopause. Magnet therapy and dietary adjustments can be safely used to address the diverse symptoms of premenstrual syndrome and menopause, as well as diseases of the uterus, vagina, bladder, and breasts.

Sore Areas in the Breast

A physician should immediately examine any sore areas in the breasts. If diagnosed as non-cancerous, you can magnetically treat the area with a 5" x 6" or 5" x 12" double magnet, multi-magnet flexible mat. On top of this mat, place a disc magnet directly over the area of soreness. Use either a 1½" x ⅛" ceramic disc magnet or a 1" x ⅛" neodymium disc magnet, held in place with a 4" x 52" body wrap or bra. Treatment should last as long as possible and should be used especially during sleep.

As a cancer preventive measure, women who know they are genetically prone to breast cancer should wear magnets over their breasts every night. As previously mentioned, the more comfortable magnets are the double magnet, multi-magnet flexible mats; either the 5" x 6" or 5" x 12" mats can be used. In addition, the mat can be reinforced with another suitably sized magnet; either a 1½" x ½" ceramic disc or a 1" x ⅛" neodymium disc magnet can be placed on top of the mat.

For more about **magnet therapy and cancer**, see Cancer.

Candidiasis (Yeast Infection)

A weak immune system as well as the intake of too many antibiotics can compromise the health of the intestinal environment. If this occurs, then the opportunistic yeast *Candida albicans* will proliferate. At this point, *Candida* becomes pathogenic, transforming from a simple yeast into an aggressive fungus that can infect other body tissues. This condition is known as candidiasis or infectious yeast overgrowth.

Candidiasis can be treated successfully with magnet therapy. Jane, for example, had candidiasis of the vagina. She obtained relief of her symptoms by sitting on the negative field side of a 4" x 6" x ½" ceramic magnet during the day, causing the fungal infection to die out. Susan had a serious case of candidiasis of the vagina and colon as well as a bacterial bladder infection. She used a 4" x 6" x ½" ceramic magnet: she sat on the negative field side of this magnet several times during the day for a total of two hours. Since beginning the magnetic therapy, no recurrence of candidiasis or infection has occurred.

For more about **magnet therapy and infections**, see Infections.

Menstrual Problems

The reproductive organs mature during puberty, the stage during which a girl becomes a woman and menstruation begins. A woman menstruates an average of 500 times during her life. Yet there are many misconceptions about menstruation, and some have been repeated so often that they are considered fact. Most notable is the assumption that the average menstrual cycle is 28 days, neatly paralleling the cycles of the moon. While women's bodies do have an observable rhythm, the menstrual cycle actually has a wide range of lengths that can be considered normal. Says Toni Weschler, M.P.H., of Seattle, Washington, "The 28-day cycle is a complete myth. Cycles vary anywhere from about 24 to 37 days. If a woman uses the 28-day cycle as a point of reference and her cycle is different," Weschler notes, "she may think there's something wrong with her."

In the early years following puberty, it is common for menstrual periods to vary due to hormonal imbalances. However, if symptoms such as irregular bleeding, midcycle spotting, bleeding with a lot of clots, or bleeding too much or too little, persist, they are signs that a woman's reproductive system needs attention. If untreated (that is, if the underlying imbalances producing them are not addressed), they can develop into full-blown conditions such as menorrhagia (excess

The Monthly Cycle

The monthly menstrual cycle results from coordinated hormonal interplay among the hypothalamus, the pituitary gland, and the ovaries. Each month, at the start of the cycle, estrogen is secreted by the ten to 20 eggs growing in the ovaries. The estrogen triggers the thickening of the lining of the uterus (the endometrium) with blood vessels, glands, and cells in anticipation of new life, and causes a fertile cervical fluid to be produced. This opens up the cervical opening to sperm and enhances the sperms' survival.

Once the mature egg has left the ovaries, it can be fertilized in the fallopian tubes. Next, estrogen production subsides and progesterone production increases. This second hormone forms a thick cervical mucous plug in the cervix to prevent sperm or bacteria from entering, and maintains the endometrium in a nutritious, blood-rich stage in anticipation of the egg's fertilization by the sperm, i.e., conception.

If conception does not occur, all hormone levels drop, some of the endometrial layer is released, or "shed," and this is called menstruation. The cycle then starts over.

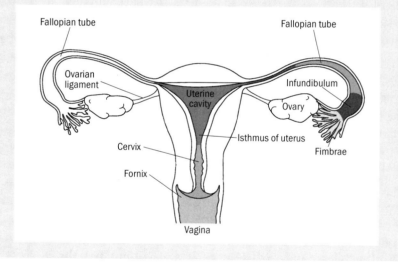

menstrual bleeding) or amenorrhea (lack of menses). New symptoms or previously only annoying symptoms may become the more serious dysmenorrhea (cramping pains with menstruation) or premenstrual syndrome (PMS) and make a woman's menstrual life miserable.

Sleeping on a magnetic bed pad with four 4" x 6" x 1" ceramic magnets at the crown of the head often relieves menstrual irregularities and related symptoms. Menstrual cramps have been successfully treated by placing a 4" x 6" x ½" magnet directly over the cramping area. You can also use a double magnet, multi-magnet flexible mat, or a 4" x 12" plastiform magnet across the abdomen. If this type of magnetic treatment is not successful, then add a 4" x 6" x $1/2$" ceramic magnet centered on top of the mat.

Menopausal Discomforts

Strictly defined, menopause is the end of all menstrual bleeding. Generally, women experience menopause between age 48 to 52, but some women cease menstruating as early as their late thirties and early forties while others stop in their mid-fifties. The aging Baby Boom population means that 3,500 American women enter the "menopausal years" every day. Yet, because women are healthier now, menopause no longer indicates the onset of old age, and women can expect to live one-third of their adult lives after menopause.[1]

Menopause is caused by the ovaries no longer producing estrogen. Perimenopause is the period before menopause, which occurs approximately between the ages of 35 to 50, but is more commonly thought of as the five to ten years before menopause. It is characterized by several years of irregular cycles with no ovulation since the ovaries are at the end of their egg supply. Without an egg's presence, progesterone is no longer produced and therefore perimenopause is frequently characterized by estrogen dominance, with side effects ranging from water retention, weight gain, and mood swings, to fibrocystic breasts, fibroids, or endometrial cancer.

Discomforts of menopause, including hot flashes, night sweats, insomnia, poor memory or poor concentration, depression, and anxiety, can be relieved with magnetic field treatment. Sleep on a magnetic bed pad with four 4" x 6" x 1" ceramic magnets at the crown of the head at night. A 30- to 60-minute bitemporal placement of $1/2$" x $3/8$" ceramic discs is also useful. This combination of magnets often relieves symptoms within minutes.

General Recommendations for Menopause

The goal of any menopausal health program should be twofold: to eliminate the bothersome symptoms of menopause and to prevent the degenerative ailments—osteoporosis and heart disease—that are associated with the postmenopausal period.

Diet—In various societies, older women traditionally eat certain foods to remedy menopausal side effects. In the South Seas, for example, once a day women of menopausal age eat papaya, which contains phytoestrogens. Studies are beginning to show that these plant compounds can be helpful in menopause.[2]

Traditional diets in Japan also are rich in phytoestrogens.[3] According to Fredi Kronenberg, Ph.D., "Studies of Japanese women with traditional Japanese diets show that these women's bodies contain levels of plant estrogens 100 to 1,000 times the level found in Western women. It may be that the reason these women don't have hot flashes is that they are eating a lot of weakly estrogenic substances all the time." She continues, "These women also have less incidence of breast cancer, and one of the reasons that is being suggested for this is that there are other things in the plant foods that are anticarcinogenic." In these studies, the higher estrogen levels were associated with intake of soybeans, soy products such as tofu and miso, and boiled beans.[4]

Legumes are an excellent source of minerals needed by postmenopausal women, containing calcium, magnesium, and potassium. They are also high in iron and in B complex, nutrients important for the health of the liver, which plays a role in the metabolism of estrogen. Seeds and nuts are also good sources of calcium, magnesium, and potassium, and seeds such as flaxseed are mildly estrogenic.

Seeds are also high in essential fatty acids. A deficiency of these oils may be responsible in part for the drying of the skin, hair, vaginal tissues, and other mucous membranes that occur with menopause; good sources are flaxseeds and pumpkin seeds.

Foods to avoid include most dairy products because of their high protein and fat content, caffeine because it can bring on hot flashes and mood swings, and alcohol because it can also lead to hot flashes. Clinical studies have shown the ability of bioflavonoids to control hot flashes.[5] Unlike estrogen therapy, no harmful side effects have been noted with bioflavonoid therapy. Vitamin E, calcium, magnesium, potassium, and aspartate may also be beneficial. Evening primrose oil is a good source of essential fatty acids.

Osteoporosis

Osteoporosis is the loss of bone density. In addition to the therapies discussed with menopause above, areas of decreased density should be treated with a negative magnetic field, which pulls minerals into the bones. It is important to use the type of magnet that penetrates deeply into the body, preferably the 4" x 6" x ½" or 4" x 6" x 1" ceramic magnets. Place directly over the affected bone. Furthermore, sleep on a magnetic bed pad with four 4" x 6" x 1" magnets at the crown of the head.

Cystitis

Cystitis refers to irritations or bacterial infections that occur anywhere in the lining of the urethra or the lining of the bladder. These infections can occur in a single episode or can exist as chronic conditions. Cystitis is common in sexually active women, and women in menopause have a tendency to develop cystitis because, as estrogen levels decline, bacteria is more prone to adhere to the bladder lining and vaginal tissue.

Symptoms include burning and pain on urination, increased urinary urgency and frequency, pain over the pubic area or lower back, and increased urination throughout the night. In women, as severity increases, blood may color the urine red. Signs that the kidneys have also become involved are fever, chills, nausea, vomiting, and severe high back and/or loin pain. For this, a doctor must be seen.

For more about **magnet therapy and infections,** see Infections.

When treating a urinary bladder infection, place a 5" x 12" double magnet, multi-magnet flexible mat across the low abdomen-pubic area. Directly on top of this mat, place a 4" x 6" x ½" magnet so it is over the bladder. This arrangement of magnets can be held in place with a 4" x 52" body wrap and should be worn as much as possible. Treatment should continue for a minimum of ten days.

Diet—"If you have an infection, taking cranberry juice, which contains hippuronic acid, makes as much sense as putting out a fire with gasoline," states Larrian Gillespie, M.D. "It only adds more acid to the urine, which in turn, increases the burning sensation. Cranberry juice may be helpful if you want to prevent an infection, but if you already have one, it only makes matters worse. Rather, try one-quarter teaspoon of baking soda in water. You should feel the relief in twenty minutes."

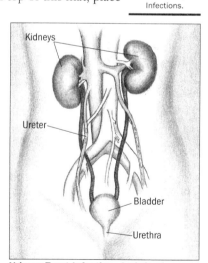

Urinary Tract Infection. An infection can develop anywhere in the urinary tract from the urethra to the kidneys. In most cases, however, the problem starts in the urethra and only moves further up the system in severe cases.

Kidneys

Ureter

Bladder

Urethra

Corn silk tea contains silica which also acts as a soothing coating to inflamed bladder tissue.

Foods which are high in the amino acids phenylalanine, tryptophan, tyrosine, and tyramine can irritate the bladder of patients with hypersensitive symptoms, adds Dr. Gillespie. Try avoiding bananas, cranberries, pineapple, avocados, aspartame, figs, yogurt, chocolate, and the citrus fruits.

Appendix

The Four-Day Rotation Diet

In spite of the knowledge of the role of maladaptive reactions to foods and the role of addictions to foods, many popular diets ignore their significance. Diets that do not treat food addictions can drive a person into the early stages of diabetes, such as hypo- or hyperglycemia. The Four-Day Diversified Rotation Diet, with the help of magnets, can relieve symptoms and help you overcome a food addiction.

It is possible to become addicted to any food eaten as frequently as twice a week. Narcotic addiction refers to being addicted to such substances as cocaine, morphine, or heroin. When exposed to a narcotic, the person feels physically and mentally euphoric, pain-free, and concern-free. Three to four hours after exposure, a withdrawal phase sets in. The body manufactures endogenous, self-made narcotics (neurotransmitters called endorphins) in response to the external narcotic, which are just as addictive. Withdrawal occurs when there is a drop in the levels of either the narcotic substance or the endorphins. The person becomes depressed, weak, agitated, or experiences pain.

All narcotics, whether produced in the body or taken externally, are alkaloids. As such, they initially raise the body's pH to an alkaline state, to make oxygen available. However, when the withdrawal phase sets in, a combination of high acidity and low levels of oxygen occurs. Addictions are thus characterized by a seesaw effect between these states of alkaline-hyperoxia and acid-hypoxia. Withdrawal symptoms develop as a result of too much acidity and low oxygen levels (acid-hypoxia) in the body. The negative magnetic field can reverse this undesirable metabolic state and change it into a more health-promoting state that supplies alkalinity and oxygen to all cells.

The addictive process also produces positive magnetic field stimulation of the brain and body. Stress is relieved by the release of serotonin and endorphins, natural opiates produced by the body. But in a state of chronic stress, the body is no longer able to produce enough serotonin or endorphins. This sets the stage for food addictions.

Foods are eaten that trigger the release of the serotonin, but at levels higher than normal, often leading to higher blood sugar levels and impaired mental functioning. Foods are thus being used as a drug to relieve symptoms and, like a drug, you can become addicted to them. This metabolic roller coaster of addiction leads to an eventual burnout of metabolic functions and a collapse of health. Fortunately,

THE FOUR-DAY ROTATION DIET

this metabolic overdrive can be reduced with sufficient negative magnetic field exposure, which normalizes the functions of the body and brain. In particular, a negative magnetic field helps to stop the addictive craving for a particular narcotic substance or food and helps to relieve withdrawal symptoms.

Gluten is the most frequent and severe symptom reactor of all foods; that is, the most likely food substance to continue evoking symptoms. Common physical reactions to gluten include such gastrointestinal problems as Celiac disease and Crohn's disease. Gluten can also cause Tourette's syndrome and severe headaches. Emotional and mental symptoms caused by reactions to gluten range from mild tension, anxiety, phobias, depression, obsessions, and compulsions to severe psychotic depression, hallucinations, and delusions. Wheat, rye, oats, and barley all contain gluten. If gluten is introduced, only a small amount should be used and then avoided for months.

In addition to being the most reactive food substance in terms of immunologic and non-immunologic maladaptive reactions, gluten is the most addictive of all food substances. Gluten is split in half during the first

Observed Facts About Maladaptive Reactions to Foods

- IgG immune food reactions are eliminated after three months of avoidance.
- Food addictions typically entail relief of symptoms on contact followed 3-4 hours later by a withdrawal phase.
- A five-day period of avoidance breaks the addiction cycle.
- The biological response to the addictive withdrawal phase is acid-hypoxia.
- Maladaptive food reactions when extended over time become chronic, degenerative diseases.

stage of digestion in the stomach, and a combination of hydrochloric acid and the enzyme pepsin accomplishes this digestive task. The splitting of gluten produces an active narcotic called exorphin. This internal narcotic is addictive when it is absorbed through the small intestine. Thus, people who are subject to gluten intolerance may experience addiction if they eat gluten-bearing foods too frequently.

Alcoholics using alcohol products prepared from wheat, rye, oats, or barley will have symptoms emerge on deliberate food testing for these gluten-containing foods. Vodka addicts have symptoms to provocative food testing for white potatoes. Wine addicts have symptoms to a provocative test meal of either grapes or the substance from which the wine is made (this applies to wine vinegar as well). Beer addicts have symptoms with test meals to brewer's yeast or any gluten-containing cereal or rice used in the beer-making process.

Dairy products and beef are the second most symptom reactive foods. Characteristically, the person who reacts to dairy products also reacts to beef, and vice versa. In terms of the frequency of symptoms, corn products are approximately equal to dairy products and beef.

Although a rotation diet solves most food reaction symptoms, there are other causes of food reactions that must sometimes be considered. Laboratory tests can make the specific determination in such cases. Diabetics on insulin, seizure cases, and dangerously aggressive psychotics should not undergo deliberate food testing without medical supervision. However, they can proceed to the rotation diet without food testing. In addition, although I do not recommend self-help food testing, its principles are as follows:

1) Maintain five days of avoidance of foods used as frequently as two or more times per week. Wait five days before using any of these foods in a single food test meal. A watermelon or water fast is best.

2) Use test meals of single foods.

3) Monitor for the emergence of physical and emotional symptoms, as well as blood pressure, both before and one hour after the meal. In addition, take the pulse before and one hour after the test meal. In the case of a non-insulin-dependent Type II diabetic, test the blood sugar before and one hour after the meal. Since many patients who have not been diagnosed as diabetic have high blood sugars beyond 160, it is a good precaution for anyone to test their blood sugar levels.

4) Use bitemporal placement of $1^1/_2$" x $^1/_2$" ceramic disc magnets to relieve mental symptoms. Hold these magnets in place with a 2" x 26" headband (see the chapter on Addictions for more details about magnetic symptom relief).

5) Stop all tobacco, alcohol, and caffeine intake when the program starts.

The Rotation Diet

Many people find it practical to implement a Four-Day Diversified Rotation Diet without having food testing done at a clinic. In order to do so, one must assume that any food, or any food-member of a particular family of foods, that is eaten as frequently as twice a week might cause a maladaptive food reaction (see "Food Family Chart," p. 222). With this assumption in mind, the individual must omit these frequently eaten foods from the diet for three months.

At the initiation of the rotation diet, the individual must also stop all use of caffeine (coffee, teas with caffeine, cola drinks, chocolate), tobacco, and alcoholic drinks, and it is important not to reintroduce these into the diet. Carbonated soft drinks are acid and should be used only rarely.

For the next three to four days, there might be withdrawal symptoms. Control of these symptoms should be managed with magnet therapy. Any specific reactive food should be brought back into the diet after three months of avoidance. At that time, 95% of the reactive foods will no longer be reactive as long as they are eaten only on a once-in-four-day basis. When reintroducing foods into the diet, simply add the food to the established rotation and observe whether or not symptoms occur. If no symptoms occur, then this food can be rotated. If symptoms occur, wait another three months before trying this food again.

For more about **magnet therapy and withdrawal symptoms**, see Addictions.

This diet selectively rotates, on a four-day basis, the foods that testing has shown to evoke symptoms. Foods that don't produce symptoms (or hypoglycemia) can be used freely at any time. One problem with this diet is that you may become addicted to some of the frequently eaten foods. Periodic food testing will alleviate this problem.

Your own rotation diet may differ from the following sample, since it should contain foods to which you are not symptom reactive. It is advisable to eat a variety of foods every day. You may move a food from one day to another (for example, if you like peas and rice together), but be careful not to repeat the same food two days in a row.

Vegetarians or others who are not consuming any animal products find it more difficult to maintain a rotation diet. One solution is to sprout cereal grains, such as wheat, rye, oats, barley, and beans. The sprouts can be considered a different food than the mature grains and can be rotated two days afterward. When sprouting grains, be sure there is about 1/4" of sprout.

Reading food labels is important so that you don't inadvertantly eat a food to which you are reactive. It is recommended that you consult your physician or health-care practitioner for further guidance.

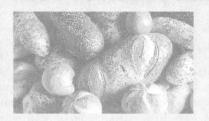

Day One

Meat/Fish: Lamb, beef, milk, yogurt, goat, deer, cheese; abalone, snail, squid, clams, mussels, oysters, scallops

Vegetables: Potato, tomato, eggplant, peppers (red/green), pimento; beets, spinach, Swiss chard, lamb's quarters; lettuce, chicory, endive, escarole, artichoke, dandelion, safflower

Fruits: Mulberry, figs, breadfruit; strawberry, raspberry, blackberry, dewberry, loganberry, youngberry, boysenberry, rose hip; grapes, raisins; mango

Nuts: Sunflower seeds; cashew, pistachio; macadamia nut

Thickening: Tapioca

Seasonings: Cream of tartar; chili pepper, paprika, cayenne; tarragon; nutmeg, mace

Oil: Safflower

Sweetener: Beet sugar

Tea: Rose hip, chicory, dandelion

Grains: None

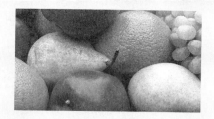

Day Two

Meat/Fish: All fowl, including chicken, turkey, duck, goose, guinea, pigeon, quail, pheasant (duck, chicken, and turkey are separate families and may be eaten every second or third day); eggs; sea herring, anchovy, cod, sea bass, sea trout, mackerel, tuna, swordfish, flounder, sole, halibut, grouper, red snapper, haddock, orange roughy

Vegetables: Pimento; millet; carrots, parsnip, celery; mushrooms, yeast (brewer's or baker's); okra

Fruits: Plum, cherry, peach, apricot, nectarine, wild cherry; pineapple; papaya, papain

Nuts: Almond; chestnut; Brazil nut; flaxseed

Thickening: Wheat flour, agar-agar (vegetable gelatin from sea algae)

Seasonings: Guava, clover, allspice, clove; celery seed, celeriac, anise, dill, fennel, cumin, parsley, coriander, caraway; sesame; vanilla

Oil: Cottonseed, flaxseed, sesame

Sweetener: Cane sugar, clover honey, molasses

Tea: Papaya tea

Grains: Wheat, oats, barley, rye; sprouts from millet, sorghum, bamboo shoot, or malt

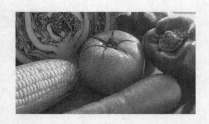

Day Three

Meat/Fish: Crab, crayfish, lobster, prawn, shrimp; pork

Vegetables: Peas, black-eyed pea, green beans, bean sprouts, soy-bean, lentil, peanut, alfalfa, lima bean, navy bean, garbanzo bean, great northern bean, pinto bean, kidney bean; avocado; onion, garlic, asparagus, chive, leek

Fruits: Apple, pear, quince; banana, plantain; blueberry, huckle-berry, cranberry; currant, gooseberry; persimmon; rhubarb

Nuts: Peanuts; filbert, hazelnut; pine nut

Thickening: Arrowroot flour

Seasonings: Arrowroot; wintergreen; licorice; cinnamon, bay leaf, sassafras, cassia bud/bark; black or white pepper

Oil: Soybean, peanut, avocado

Sweetener: Fructose, carob syrup, maple sugar, tupelo honey

Tea: Alfalfa, sassafras, garlic, apple cider/tea

Grains: Buckwheat, rice

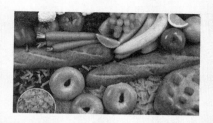

Day Four

Meat/Fish: Rabbit; fowl not used on day two (chicken, turkey, duck); sturgeon, herring, salmon, whitefish, bass, perch, and any fresh-water fish

Vegetables: Sweet potato; cucumber, pumpkin, squash, zucchini, acorn, pumpkin, squash seeds; mustard, turnip, radish, horseradish, watercress, cabbage, kraut, Chinese cabbage, broccoli, cauliflower, Brussels sprouts, collard, kale, kohlrabi, rutabaga; black/green olives; fresh corn, hominy, grits

Fruits: Watermelon, cantaloupe, honeydew; lemon, orange, grapefruit, lime, tangerine, kumquat, citron; elderberry; coconut, date

Nuts: Pumpkin seeds, squash seeds, coconut; English walnut, black walnut, pecan, hickory, butternut

Thickening: Cornstarch

Seasonings: Mustard; basil, sage, oregano, savory horehound, catnip, spearmint, peppermint, thyme, marjoram, lemon balm

Oil: Coconut, olive, pecan, corn

Sweetener: Date sugar, honey (other than tupelo or clover), corn sugar

Tea: Kaffer

Grains: None

Food Family Chart

Meat: beef, cow's milk, goat's milk, pork, lamb

Fowl: chicken, turkey, duck, goose, eggs,

Freshwater fish: bass, perch, pike, salmon, trout

Saltwater fish: anchovy, cod, eel, herring, mackerel, mullet, sardine, sole, tuna

Crustacean: crab, lobster, shrimp

Mollusks: clams, mussels, oyster, scallop

Grass: barley, corn, kamut, malt, millet, oat, quinoa, rice, rye, spelt, wheat, wild rice

Legumes: beans, lentil, peanut, peas, soybean, tamarind, alfalfa sprouts, licorice, carob

Mustard greens: broccoli, Brussels sprout, cabbage, cauliflower, horseradish, kale, kohlrabi, mustard greens, mustard seed, radish, turnip, watercress

Parsley: anise, caraway, carrot, celery, celeriac, chervil, coriander, cumin, dill, lovage, parsley, parsnip

Potato: cayenne, chili pepper, eggplant, paprika, peppers, potatoes, white potatoes, tobacco

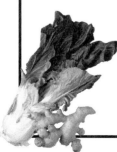

Lily: asparagus, chive, garlic, leek, onion

Sunflower (aster): artichoke, chicory, endive, Jerusalem artichoke, dandelion, tarragon, chamomile, sunflower, safflower, yarrow

Beet: beet, chard, spinach, sugar beet

Buckwheat: buckwheat, rhubarb, sorrel

Laurel: avocado, camphor, cinnamon, bay leaf

Melon: cantaloupe, cucumber, honeydew, pumpkin, squash, zucchini

Plum: almond, apricot, cherry, nectarine, peach, plum

Citrus: citron, grapefruit, lemon, lime, orange, tangerine

Banana: arrowroot, banana, plantain

Palm: coconut, date, date sugar

Grape: grape, raisin, cream of tartar

Rose: blackberry, loganberry, raspberry, rosehip, strawberry

Apple: apple, loquat, pear, quince

Blueberry: blueberry, cranberry, huckleberry

Cashew: cashew, mango, pistachio

Nuts: Brazil nut, pecan, walnut

Beech: beechnut, chestnut

Birch: filbert, hazelnut

Walnut: butternut, hickory nut, pecan, walnut

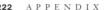

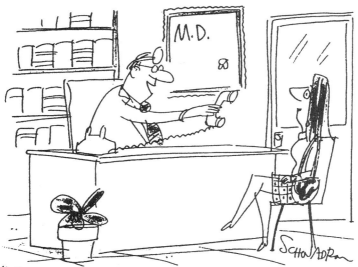

" I NOW OFFER NUTRITIONAL COUNSELING. HERE'S A RECORDING OF MY MOM'S RECIPE FOR CHICKEN SOUP. "

Endnotes

Chapter I
What is Magnet Therapy?

1 R.O. Becker, M.D. *Cross Currents* (Los Angeles: Jeremy P. Tarcher, 1990).

2 Ron Lawrence, M.D., Ph.D. and Paul J. Rosch, M.D., F.A.C.P. *Magnet Therapy: The Pain Cure Alternative* (Rocklin, CA: Prima Health, 1998), 38.

3 George J. Washnis and Richard Z. Hricak. *Discovery of Magnetic Health* (Rockville, MD: Nova Publishing, 1993), 8.

4 Cyril W. Smith and Simon Best. *Electromagnetic Man* (London: J.M. Dent and Sons, 1989), 8-9.

5 Y. Aharonov and D. Bohn. "Significance of Electromagnetic Potentials in Quantum Theory." *The Physical Revision* 115 (1959), 485. In 1986, Aharonov-Rolm effect was confirmed by Akaira Tonomura at Hitachi, Ltd., in Tokyo.

6 R.O. Becker and G. Seldon. *The Body Electric: ElectroMagnetism and the Foundation of Life* (New York: William Marrow, 1986).

7 "Electricity and Magnetism." *Encyclopedia Britannica* Vol. 18 15th Ed. (Chicago: Encyclopedia Britannica, 1991), 175.

8 Ibid.

9 R.O. Becker, M.D. *Cross Currents* (Los Angeles: Jeremy P. Tarcher, 1990).

10 *New Encyclopedia* Vol. 24 (Chicago: Encyclopedia Britannica, 1986), 200.

11 Philip Callahan. *Ancient Mysteries, Modern Visions: The Magnetic Life of Agriculture* (Kansas City, MO: Acres USA, 1984).

12 Kyoichi Nakagawa. "Magnetic Field Deficiency Syndrome and Magnetic Treatment." *Japanese Medical Journal* 2715 (December 4, 1976).

13 N. Wertheimer and E. Leeper. "Electrical Wiring Configurations and Childhood Cancer." *American Journal of Epidemiology* 109 (1979), 273-284.

14 J. Wolpay. *Biological Effects of Power Line Fields* (New York: New York State Power-Lines Project Scientific Advisory Panel, 1987).

15 M. Speers, J. Dobbins, and V. Miller. "Occupational Exposures and Brain Cancer Mortality: A Preliminary Study of East Texas Residents." *American Journal of Industrial Medicine* 13 (198), 629-638.

16 R.O. Becker, M.D. *Cross Currents* (Los Angeles: Jeremy P. Tarcher, 1990), 208.

17 Cyril W. Smith and Simon Best. *Electromagnetic Man* (London: J.M. Dent and Sons, 1989).

18 J.C. Murphy et al. "Power Frequency Electric and Magnetic Fields: A Review of Genetic Toxicology." *Mutation Research* 296:3 (March 1993), 221-240.

19 R.O. Becker, M.D. *Cross Currents* (Los Angeles: Jeremy P. Tarcher, 1990), 210.

20 J. Fontenot and S.A. Levine. "Melatonin Deficiency: Its Role in Oncogenesis and Age-Relative Pathology." *Journal of Orthomolecular Medicine* 5:1 (1990), 22-24.

21 A.R. Davis and W.C. Rawls. *Magnetism and Its Effects of the Living System* (New York: Exposition Press, 1974).

22 Ron Lawrence, M.D., Ph.D., Paul J. Rosch, M.D., F.A.C.P., and Judith Plowden. *Magnet Therapy: The Pain Cure Alternative* (Rocklin, CA: Prima Health, 1998), 2.

23 Julian Whitaker, M.D., and Brenda Adderly, M.H.A. *The Pain Relief Breakthrough* (Boston: Little, Brown,

and Co., 1998), 22.

24 Ron Lawrence, M.D., Ph.D., Paul J. Rosch, M.D., F.A.C.P., and Judith Plowden. *Magnet Therapy: The Pain Cure Alternative* (Rocklin, CA: Prima Health, 1998), 6. Julian Whitaker, M.D., and Brenda Adderly, M.H.A. *The Pain Relief Breakthrough* (Boston: Little, Brown, and Co., 1998), 23-25.

25 Ron Lawrence, M.D., Ph.D., Paul J. Rosch, M.D., F.A.C.P., and Judith Plowden. *Magnet Therapy: The Pain Cure Alternative* (Rocklin, CA: Prima Health, 1998), 12.

26 Julian Whitaker, M.D., and Brenda Adderly, M.H.A. *The Pain Relief Breakthrough* (Boston: Little, Brown, and Co., 1998), 23.

27 Ron Lawrence, M.D., Ph.D., Paul J. Rosch, M.D., F.A.C.P., and Judith Plowden. *Magnet Therapy: The Pain Cure Alternative* (Rocklin, CA: Prima Health, 1998), 13-17.

28 Ibid., 20-21.

29 "Electricity and Magnetism." *Encyclopedia Britannica* Vol. 18 15th Ed. (Chicago: Encyclopedia Britannica, 1991), 189-193.

30 Julian Whitaker, M.D., and Brenda Adderly, M.H.A. *The Pain Relief Breakthrough* (Boston: Little, Brown, and Co., 1998), 36-37.

Chapter 2

How Magnets Heal

1 R.O. Becker and A.A. Marino. *Electromagnetism & Life.* (Albany, NY: State University of New York Press, 1982). R.O. Becker and G. Seldon. *The Body Electric: Electromagnetism & the Foundation of Life* (New York: William Morrow, 1986).

2 R.O. Becker. *Cross Currents* (Los Angeles: Jeremy P. Tarcher, 1990), 77.

3 J. Fontenot and S.A. Levine. "Melatonin Deficiency: Its Role in Oncogenesis and Age-Relative Pathology." *Journal of Orthomolecular Medicine* 5:1 (1990).

4 G.H. Daniels and J.B. Martin. *Harrison's Principles of Internal Medicine* 11th ed. (New York; McGraw-Hill, 1987), 1701-1705.

5 R.O. Becker and A.A. Marino. *Electromagnetism & Life* (Albany, NY: University of New York Press, 1982). R.O. Becker and G. Seldon. *The Body Electric* (New York: William Morrow, 1986). R.O. Becker. *Cross Currents* (Los Angeles: Jeremy P. Tarcher, 1990).

6 J. Jerabek and W. Pawluk. *Magnetic Therapy in Eastern Europe: A Review of 30 Years of Research* (Chicago: William Pawluk, M.D., 1998). C. Polk and E. Postow, eds. *Handbook of Biological Effects of Electromagnetic Fields* 2nd ed. (Boca Raton, FL: CRC Press, 1996).

7 J. Jerabek and W. Pawluk. *Magnetic Therapy in Eastern Europe: A Review of 30 Years of Research* (Chicago: William Pawluk, M.D., 1998). U. Warnke. "Infrared Radiation and Oxygen Partial Pressure in Human Surfacial Tissue as Indicators of the Therapeutic Effects of Pulsating Magnetic Fields of Extremely Low Frequency." *Biophysical Medicine Report* 2 (1981), 1-8.

8 K. Vrecko, J.G.D. Birkmayer, and J. Krainz. "Stimulation of Dopamine Biosynthesis in Cultured PC12 Phaeochromocytoma Cells by the Coenzyme Nicotinamide Adenine Dinucleotide (NADH)." *Journal of Neural Transmission* 5 (1993), 147-156. J.G.D. Birkmayer. "Nicotinamide Adenine Dinucleotide (NADH): The New Therapeutic Approach for Improving Dementia of the Alzheimer Type." *Annals of Clinical and Laboratory Science* (Unpublished manuscript). J.G.D. Birkmayer et al. "Nicotinamide Adenine Dinucleotide (NADH): A New Therapeutic Approach to Parkinson's Disease: Comparison of

Oral and Parenteral Application." *Acta Neurologica Scandinavica* 87:Suppl 146 (1993), 32-35. W. Birkmayer and J.G.D. Birkmayer. "Nicotinamide Adenine Dinucleotide (NADH) as Medication for Depressed Patients: Experience With 205 Patients." *New Trends in Clinical Neuropharmacology* 5 (1991), 15-23.

9 R.A. Passwater, Ph.D. *Lipoic Acid: The Metabolic Antioxidant Good Health Guide* (New Canaan, CT: Keats Publishing, 1995).

10 J. Jerabek and W. Pawluk. *Magnetic Therapy in Eastern Europe: A Review of 30 Years of Research* (Chicago: William Pawluk, M.D., 1998). J. Walleczek. "Magnetokinetic Effects on Radical Pairs: A Paradigm for Magnetic Field Interactions with Biologic Systems at Lower Than Thermal Energy." In: M. Blank, ed. *Electromagnetic Fields: Biological Interactions and Mechanisms* (Washington, DC: American Chemical Society, 1995).

11 R. Becker. *Cross Currents* (Los Angeles: Jeremy P. Tarcher, 1990), 77.

12 G.H. Daniels and J.B. Martin. *Harrison's Principles of Internal Medicine* 11th ed. (New York: McGraw-Hill, 1987), 1701-1705.

13 J. Jerabek and W. Pawluk. *Magnetic Therapy in Eastern Europe: A Review of 30 Years of Research* (Chicago: William Pawluk, M.D., 1998). R.B. Frankel and R.P. Liburdy. "Biological Effects of Static Magnetic Fields." In: C. Polk and E. Postow, eds. *Handbook of Biological Effects of Electromagnetic Fields* 2nd ed. (Boca Raton, FL: CRC Press, 1996).

Chapter 3

Magnet Therapy in Practice

1 Ron Lawrence, M.D., Ph.D., and Paul J. Rosch, M.D., F.A.C.P. *Magnet Therapy: The Pain Cure Alternative* (Rocklin, CA: Prima Publishing, 1998), 117.

An A-Z of Health Conditions

Alzheimer's Disease

1 D.A. Evans, M.D., et al. "Prevalence of Alzheimer's Disease in a Community Population of Older Persons: Higher than Previously Reported." *Journal of the American Medical Association* 262:18 (November 1989), 2551-2556.

2 W. Klonowski and M. Klonowski. "Aging Process and Enzymatic Proteins," *Journal of Bioelectricity* 4 (1) (1985): 93-102.

3 William H. Philpott and Dwight K. Kalita. *Victory Over Diabetes: A Bio-Ecologic Triumph* (New Canaan, CT: Keats Publishing, 1983).

4 D.M Mann and M.M. Esiri. "The Pattern of Acquisition of Plaques and Tangles in the Brains of Patients Under 50 Years of Age with Down's Syndrome." *Journal of the Neurological Sciences* 89:2-3 (February 1989), 169-179.

5 Editorial Staff. "Growing Evidence for Aluminum/Alzheimer's Link." *Clinical Psychiatry News* (December 1988), 2.

6 Research study from the Sanders-Brown Center on Aging at the University of Kentucky Medical Center, Lexington, KY, published in *Neurotoxicology* 9 (1988), 1.

7 R. Shiele et al. "Studies on the Mercury Content in Brain and Kidney Related to Number and Condition of Dental Fillings." Institution of Occupational and Social Medicine, University Erlangen, Nurnberg, West Germany (March 12, 1984).

8 M. Fisman. *American Journal of Psychiatry* 142 (1985), 71-73.

9 M.R. Werbach, M.D. *Nutritional Influences on Mental Illness* (Tarzana, CA: Third Line Press, 1993). D.C. Martin. "B12 and Folate Deficiency Dementia." *Clinics in Geriatric Medicine* 4:4 (November 1988), 841-

852. D.E. Thomas et al. "Tryptophan and Nutritional Status of Patients with Senile Dementia." *Psychological Medicine* 16:2 (May 1986), 297-305. A.M. Keatinge et al. "Vitamin B1, B2, B6 and C Status in the Elderly." *Irish Medical Journal* 76 (December 1983), 488-490. G.E. Gibson et al. "Reduced Activities of Thiamine-Dependent Enzymes in the Brains and Peripheral Tissues of Patients with Alzheimer's Disease." *Archives of Neurology* 45:8 (August 1988), 836-840. M.G. Cole and J.F. Prchal. "Low Serum B12 in Alzheimer-Type Dementia." *Age and Ageing* 13:2 (Mar,1984): 101-5. Burns, A; and Holland, T. "Vitamin E Deficiency." *The Lancet* 1:8484 (April 1986), 805-806. I.J. Deary et al. "Serum Calcium Levels in Alzheimer's Disease: A Finding and an Aetiological Hypothesis." *Personality and Individual Differences* 8:1 (1987), 75-80. K. Torizumi et al. "Relationship Between Parathyroid Hormone and Magnesium in Sera of Dementia Patients." *Radioisotopes* 37:4 (April 1988), 203-208. N.I. Ward and J.A. Mason. "Neutron Activation Analysis Techniques for Identifying Elemental Status in Alzheimer's Disease." *Journal of Radioanalytic Nuclear Chemistry* 113:2 (1987), 515-526.

10 George G. Glenner and Jay H. Stein. *Internal Medicine* 4th ed. (St. Louis, MO: Mosby, 1994), 2513-2514.

11 R. Sandyk. "Alzheimer's Disease: Improvement of Visual Memory and Visuoconstructive Performance by Treatment with Picotesla Range Magnetic Fields." *International Journal of Neuroscience* 76:3-4 (1994), 185-225.

12 M. Imagawa et al. "Coenzyme Q10, Iron, and Vitamin B6 in Genetically Confirmed Alzheimer's Disease." *The Lancet* 340:8820 (September 1992), 671.

13 *Journal of Nutrition Research* 1, 259-266.

14 E. McDonagh, C. Rudolph, and E. Cheraskin. "An Oculocerebro-vasculo-metric Analysis of the Improve-ment in Arterial Stenosis Following EDTA Chelation Therapy." *Journal of Advancement in Medicine* 2:1-2 (1989), 155. H.R. Casdorph. "EDTA Chelation Therapy: Efficacy in Brain Disorders." *Journal of Advancement in Medicine* 2:1-2 (1989), 131-153.

Cancer

1 J. Madeleine Nash. "The Enemy Within." *Time* (Fall 1996), 20.

2 American Cancer Society. *Facts about Cancer* (Atlanta, GA: American Cancer Society, 1996).

3 J.S. Bailar and E.M. Smith. "Progress Against Cancer?" *New England Journal of Medicine* 314 (1986), 1226.

4 B. Hankey, Chief of the Cancer Statistics Branch, National Cancer Institute. Personal communications (1994). The incidence of all cancers combined for the total population increased 13% from 1975 to 1989, from 332 per 100,000 to 376 per 100,000. The mortality rate rose 7%, from 162 deaths per 100,000 to 173 per 100,000.

5 National Cancer Institute. *Cancer Statistics Review, 1973-1989* (Washington, DC: National Institutes of Health, Office of Cancer Communications, 1992).

6 Tim Beardsley. "A War Not Won." *Scientific American* (January 1994), 130-138.

7 M. Wasserman et al. "Organochlorine Compounds in Neoplastic and Adjacent Apparently Normal Breast Tissue." *Bulletin of Environmental Contaminants and Toxicology* 15 (1976), 478-484.

8 J. Westin and E. Richter. "Israeli Breast

Cancer Anomaly." *Annals of the New York Academy of Sciences* 609 (1990), 269-279.

9 O. Warburg. *The Metabolism of Tumors*. F. Dickens (trans) (London: Arnold Constable, 1930). T.E. Tavnock and D. Rotin. "Acid pH in Tumors and Its Potential for Therapeutic Exploitation." *Cancer Research* 49 (1989). 437-438.

10 R.O. Becker and G. Seldon. *The Body Electric: Electro- Magnetism and the Foundation of Life* (New York: William Morrow, 1986). R.O. Becker. *Cross Currents* (Los Angeles: Jeremy P. Tarcher, 1990).

11 Arthur Trappier et al. "Evaluating Perspectives on the Exposure Risks from Magnetic Fields." *Journal of the National Medical Association* 82:9 (September 1990), 621-624.

12 R.R. Raylman et al., "Exposure to Strong Static Magnetic Field Slows the Growth of Human Cancer Cells in Vitro." *Bioelectromagnetics* 17:5 (1996), 358-363. N.G. Bakhmutskii et al. "The Growth Dynamics of Walker Carcinosarcoma During Exposure to a Magnetic Eddy Field." *Vopr Onkol* 37:6 (1991), 705-708.

13 N.G. Bakhmutskii et al. "The Assessment of the Efficacy of the Effect of a Rotational Magnetic Field on the Course of the Tumor Process in Patients with Generalized Breast Cancer." *Soviet Medicine* 7 (1991), 25-27.

14 M. Riviere et al. "Test with Lymphosarcoma on Mice." *Comptes Rendus de'l'Academie des Sciences* (March 1, 1965).

15 I. Troeng. Commenting on the study's results. Laholm, Sweden (July 1984). See: M. Riviere et al. "Test with Lymphosarcoma on Mice." *Comptes Rendus de'l'Academie des Sciences* (March 1, 1965).

Children's Health Problems

1 T.W. Jones et al. "Independent Effects of Youth and Poor Diabetes Control on Responses to Hypoglycemia in Children." *Diabetes* 40:3 (March 1991), 358-363.

2 J.L. Rapoport. "Diet and Hyperactivity." *Nutrition Reviews* 44:Suppl (May 1986), 158-162.

3 U.S. Department of Health and Human Services, Public Health Service. *More Than You Ever Thought You Would Know About Food Additives* (Washington, DC: Food and Drug Administration, 1982).

4 J. Egger et al. "Controlled Trial of Oligoantigenic Treatment in the Hyperkinetic Syndrome." *The Lancet* 1:8428 (March 1985), 540-545.

5 J.P. Harley et al. "Hyperkinesis and Food Additives: Testing the Feingold Hypothesis." *Pediatrics* 61:6 (1978), 818-828.

6 Consensus Conference: "Defined Diets and Childhood Hyperactivity." *Journal of the American Medical Association* 248:3 (July 1982), 29029-29032.

7 J. Egger, A. Stolla, and L.M. McEwen. "Controlled Trial of Hyposensitisation in Children with Food-Induced Hyperkinetic Syndrome." *The Lancet* 339:8802 (May 1992), 1150-1153.

Chronic Fatigue Syndrome

1 Available at the U.S Centers for Disease Control website: www.cdc.gov/nci-dod.diseases/cfs/facts.htm.

2 U.S. Centers for Disease Control. "The Facts About Chronic Fatigue Syndrome" (August 1994). Available at the U.S Centers for Disease Control website: www.cdc.gov/ncidod.dis-eases/cfs/facts.htm.

3 Jesse A. Stoff, M.D., and Charles R. Pellegrino, Ph.D. *Chronic Fatigue Syndome: The Hidden Epidemic* (New York: HarperCollins, 1992).

4 Linda Rector Page, N.D., Ph.D. *Healthy Healing* (Sonora, CA: Healthy Healing Publications, 1997), 115. Burton Goldberg and the Editors of *Alternative*

Medicine Digest. *Chronic Fatigue, Fibromyalgia, and Environment Illness* (Tiburon, CA: Future Medicine Publishing, 1998).

5 M. Rosenbaum, M.D., and M. Susser, M.D. *Solving the Puzzle of Chronic Fatigue Syndrome* (Tacoma, WA: Life Sciences Press, 1992), 44

6 T. Prince et al. "Chronic Fatigue in a 43-Year-Old Woman." *Annals of Allergy* 74 (June 1995), 474-478.

Diabetes

1 John Potts and E. Sanai. "Avoidance Provocative Food Testing in Assessing Diabetes Responsiveness." *Diabetes* 26:Suppl 1 (1977). John Potts. "Value of Specific Testing for Assessing Insulin Resistance." *Diabetes* 29:Suppl 2 (1980). John Potts. "Blood Sugar-Insulin Responses to Specific Food Viruses GTT." *Diabetes* 30:Suppl 2 (1980). John Potts. "Insulin Resistance Related to Specific Food Sensitivity." Diabetes 35:Suppl 1 (1986).

2 J.E. Pizzorno and M.T. Murray. "Diabetes Mellitus." In: J. E. Pizzorno and M. T. Murray, ed. *A Textbook of Natural Medicine* (Seattle, WA: John Bastyr College Publications, 1988).

3 Suvi M. Virtanen, M.D. "Infant Feeding of Finnish Children Up to 7 Years of Age with Newly Diagnosed IDDM." *Diabetes Care* 14:5 (May 1991). K. Jukka, M.D. "A Bovine Albumin Peptide as A Possible Trigger of Insulin-Dependent Diabetes Mellitus." *New England Journal of Medicine* 327:5 (July 30, 1992), 302-307.

4 R.L. Searcy, M.D. *Diagnostic Biochemistry* (New York: McGraw-Hill, 1969).

5 E. Albert, M.D. "Current Concepts in Diabetes Mellitus." *New York State Journal of Medicine* 53:22 (November 1953), 2607-2610.

6 J.M. Ellis, M.D. *Vitamin B6: The Doctor's Report* (New York: Harper & Row, 1973).

7 C.L. Jones and V. Gonzalez, M.D. "Pyroxidine Deficiency: A New Factor in Diabetic Neuropathy." *Journal of American Podiatry Association* 68:9 (September 1978), 646-653.

8 J.E. Pizzorno and M.T. Murray. *A Textbook of Natural Medicine* (Seattle WA: John Bastyr College Publications, 1988), 14.

9 D. Koutsikos, B. Agroyannis, and H. Tzanatos-Exarchou. "Biotin for Diabetic Peripheral Neuropathy." *Biomedicine and Pharmacotherapy* 44:10 (1990), 511-514.

10 P.S. Devamanoharan et al. "Prevention of Selenite Cataract by Vitamin C." *Experimental Eye Research* 52:5 (May 1991), 563-568.

11 W.H. Philpott and D.K. Kalita. *Victory Over Diabetes* (New Canaan, CT: Keats Publishing, 1983).

12 W.E. Shute. *Vitamin E for Ailing and Healthy Hearts* (New York: Pyramid House, 1969).

13 C. Colette et al. "Platelet Function in Type I Diabetes: Effects of Supplementation with Large Doses of Vitamin E." *American Journal of Clinical Nutrition* 47:2 (February 1988), 256-261.

14 M.J. Stuart. "Vitamin E Deficiency: its Effect on Platelet-Vascular Interaction in Various Pathological States." *Annals of the New York Academy of Sciences* 393 (1982), 277-288. J. Watanabe et al. "Effect of Vitamin E on Platelet Aggregation in Diabetes Mellitus." *Thrombosis and Haemostasis* 51 (1984), 313-316.

15 Editorial Staff. "Chromium Enrichment of Foods Urged." *Medical World News* 15:7 (October 1974), 33-35.

16 E.W. Toepfer et al. "Chromium in Foods Related to Biological Activity." *Journal of Agricultural Food Chemistry* 21:1 (1973), 69-73.

17 J.E. Pizzorno and M.T. Murray. *A Textbook of Natural Medicine* (Seattle,

WA: John Bastyr College Publications, 1988), 10-11.

18 W. Merz and K. Schwarz. 'Relation of Glucose Tolerance Factor to Impaired Intravenous Glucose Tolerance of Rats on a Stock Diet." *American Journal of Physiology* 196:3 (1959), 614-618.

19 K.M. Hambidge. "Chromium Nutrition in Man." *American Journal of Clinical Nutrition* 27:5 (May 1974), 505-514.

20 A. Sjogren et al. "Magnesium, Potassium, and Zinc Deficiencies in Subjects with Type II Diabetes." *Acta Medica Scandinavica* 224 (1988), 461-463.

21 J. Sheehan. "Importance of Magnesium Chloride Repletion after Myocardial Infarction." *American Journal of Cardiology* 63:14 (April 1989), 35G-38G.

22 R.A. Reinhart. "Clinical Correlates of the Molecular and Cellular Actions of Magnesium on the Cardiovascular System." *American Heart Journal* 121:5 (May 1991), 1513-1521.

23 G. Norbiato et al. "Effects of Potassium Supplementation on Insulin Binding and Insulin Action in Human Obesity: Protein-Modified Fast and Refeeding" *European Journal of Clinical Investigation* 14:6 (December 1984), 414-419.

24 E.J. Underwood, M.D. *Trace Elements in Human and Animal Nutrition* (Orlando, FL: Academic Press, 1986-1987).

25 K. Keeton. *Longevity: The Science of Staying Young* (New York: Viking, 1992).

26 A. Weil. *Natural Health, Natural Medicine* (Boston: Houghton Mifflin, 1990), 279.

27 W.H. Philpott, M.D., and D.K. Kalita. *Victory Over Diabetes* (New Canaan, CT: Keats Publishing, 1983).

28 G. Riccardi and A.A. Rivallese. "Effects of Dietary Fiber and Carbohydrate on Glucose and Lipoprotein Metabolism in Diabetes Patients." *Diabetes Care* 14 (December 1991), 1115-1125.

29 I.B. Kirillov et al. "Magnetotherapy in the Comprehensive Treatment of Vascular Complications of Diabetes Mellitus." *Klin Med* 74:5 (1996), 39-41.

30 R.A. Kuliev and R.F. Babaev. "A Magnetic Field in the Combined Treatment of Suppurative Wounds in Diabetes Mellitus." *Vestn Khir Im I I Grek* 148:1 (1992), 33-36.

Environmental Illness

1 William Lee Cowden, M.D., "Is Your Shower Toxic? Some Pollution Solutions." *Alternative Medicine* 29 (April/May 1999), 69.

2 B. Croty "Ulcerative Colitis and Xenobiotic Metabolism." *The Lancet* 343 (1990), 35-38.

3 William Lee Cowden, M.D., "Is Your Shower Toxic? Some Pollution Solutions." *Alternative Medicine* 29 (April/May 1999), 69.

4 W. Melillo. "How Safe is Mercury in Dentistry?" *Washington Post Weekly Journal of Medicine, Science and Society* (September 1991), 4. World Health Organization. *Environmental Health Criteria for Inorganic Mercury* (Geneva, Switzerland: World Health Organization, 1991), 118.

5 William J. Rea, M.D. *Chemical Sensitivity*, Vol. 3 (Boca Raton, FL: C.R.C. Lewis, 1996), 1555-1579.

6 D.N. Taylor et al. "Effects of Trichloroethylene in the Exploratory and Locomotor Activity in Rats Exposed During Development." *Science Total Environment* 47 (1985), 415-420. H.N. Arito, T. Suruta, K. Nakagaki, and S. Tanaka. "Partial Insomnia, Hyperactivity and Hyperdipsia Induced by Repeated Administration of Toluene in Rats: Their Relation to Brain Monoamine Metabolism." *Toxicology* 37:1-2 (1985), 99-110.

7 R. Edwards. "Leak Links Power Lines to Cancer." *New Scientist* 4 (October 7,

1995), 4.

8 C. Ezzell. "Power-Line Static. Debates Rage Over the Possible Hazards of Electromagnetic Fields." *Science News* 140 (September 1991), 202-203.

9 D. Wartenberg. "EMFs: Cutting Through the Controversy." *Public Health Reports* 111:3 (May/June 1996), 204-217.

10 Robert O. Becker, M.D. *Cross Currents: The Perils of Electropollution, The Promise of Electromedicine* (New York: Jeremy P. Tarcher, 1990), 270.

11 Michael Hodgson, M.D., M.P.H. "The Medical Evaluation" and "The Sick Building Syndrome" in Effects of the Indoor Environment on Health. Cited in: *Occupational Medicine: State of the Art Reviews* 10:1 (January-March 1995), 167-194.

Eye Disorders

1 M.A. Krupp, M.J. Chatton, and L.M. Tierney, eds. *Current Medical Diagnosis and Treatment* (Los Altos, CA: Lange Medical Publications, 1982), 77-84.

2 J.E. Pizzorno and M.T. Murray. *A Textbook of Natural Medicine* (Seattle, WA: John Bastyr College Publications, 1989).

3 A.R. Gaby, M.D., and J.V. Wright, M.D. "Nutritional Factors in Degenerative Eye Disorders: Cataract and Macular Degeneration." *Journal of Advancement in Medicine* 6:1 (Spring 1993), 27-39.

4 A.R. Gaby, M.D., and J.V. Wright, M.D. "Nutritional Factors in Degenerative Eye Disorders: Cataract and Macular Degeneration." *Journal of Advancement in Medicine* 6:1 (Spring 1993), 27-39.

Gastrointestinal Problems

1 J.E. Pizzorno and M.T. Murray. *Encyclopedia of Natural Medicine*

(Rocklin, CA: Prima Publishing, 1991), 395.

Heart Disease

1 James R. Privitera, M.D. *Clots: Life's Biggest Killer* (Unpublished manuscript).

2 S.L. Robbins, R.S. Cotran, and V. Kumar, eds. *Pathological Basis of Disease* (New York: W.B. Saunders, 1984).

3 Burton Goldberg and The Editors of Alternative Medicine. *Alternative Medicine Guide to Heart Disease* (Tiburon, CA: Future Medicine Publishing, 1998), 33.

4 Melvyn R. Werbach, M.D. *Nutritional Influences on Illness: A Sourcebook of Clinical Research* (Tarzana, CA: Third Line Press, 1988), 238-239.

5 Gary Null, Ph.D. *The Clinician's Handbook of Natural Healing* (New York: Kensington Publishing, 1997), 46-53.

6 Ibid., 286-306.

Infections

1 A. O. Davis, *The Magnetic Effect* (Kansas City, MO: Acres USA, 1975), 64.

2 Ibid.

3 J. Jung, E. Sanai, S. Godbole, & S. Sofer, "Separate Biological Responses to Opposite Magnetic Fields Demonstrated by Bacterial Culture." *News release from New Jersey Institute of Technology* (January 18, 1993).

4 *Harrison's Principles of Internal Medicine* (New York: McGraw-Hill, 1985), 1797.

Men's Health Problems

1 J.I. Silverstein, G.H. Baldini, and A.D. Smith. "Management of Benign Prostatic Hypertrophy." *Clinical Geriatric Medicine* 6, 69-84.

Mental and Emotional Problems

1 D.A. Regier et al. "The De Facto U.S. Mental and Addictive Disorders Service System." *Archives of General Psychiatry* 50 (February 1993), 85.

2 C.B. Clayman, ed. *The American Medical Association Encyclopedia of Medicine* (New York: Random House, 1989).

3 P.R. Breggin. *Toxic Psychiatry* (New York: St. Martin's Press, 1991).

4 R. Sandyk, P.A. Anninos, and N. Tsagas. "Magnetic Fields and Seasonality of Affective Illness: Implications for Therapy." *International Journal of Neuroscience* 58:3-4 (1991), 261-267.

Multiple Sclerosis

1 *Proceedings of the National Academy of Sciences* 92 (1995), 7440-7444.

2 International Labour Office. *Encyclopedia of Occupational Health and Safety* 2d ed. (New York: McGraw-Hill, 1972).

3 M.J. Vimy, Y. Takahashi, and F.L. Lorscheider. "Maternal-Fetal Distribution of Mercury Released From Dental Amalgam Fillings." *American Physiological Society* 258 (1990), R939-R945. F.L. Lorscheider, et al. "Mercury From Amalgam Tooth Fillings: Its Tissue Distribution and Effects on Cell Functions." *The Toxicologist* 12 (1992), 1.

4 M.J. Vimy et al. "Glomerular Filtration Impairment by Mercury from Dental 'Silver' Fillings in Sheep." *The Physiologist* 33 (August 1990), A 94. N.D. Boyd et al. "Mercury from Dental 'Silver' Tooth Fillings Impairs Sheep Kidney Function." *American Physiological Society* 261 (1991), R1010-R1014. B. Ahlrot-Westerlund, M.D. "Mercury in Cerebrospinal Fluid in Multiple Sclerosis." *Sweden Journal of Biological Medicine* 1 (March 1989), 6.

5 C.J. Webster et al. "The Chief Scientist Reports...Hyperbaric Oxygen for Multiple Sclerosis." *Health Bulletin* 47:6 (November 1989), 320-331.

6 M.P. Barnes et al. "Hyperbaric Oxygen and Multiple Sclerosis: Short-Term Results of a Placebo-Controlled Double-Blind Trial." *The Lancet* 1:8424 (February 1985), 287-300. C.M. Wiles et al. "Hyperbaric Oxygen in Multiple Sclerosis: A Double-Blind Trial." *British Medical Journal* 292:6517 (February 1986), 367-371.

Obesity

1 Robert J. Kuczmarski, Dr.PH., R.D., et al. "Weight Gain on the Rise in the United States." *Journal of the American Medical Association* 272:3 (1994), 205-211. F. Xavier Pi-Sunyer, M.D. "The Fattening of America." *Journal of the American Medical Association* 272:3 (1994), 238.

2 Lisa Grunwald. "Discovery: Do I look Fat to You? 28 Questions (and All the Answers) About Our National Obsession." *Life* (February 1, 1995), 58.

3 Peggy Olivero. "Obesity: The Next Generation." *Nourish* (February/March 1996, 8.

4 Michael T. Murray, N.D. *Natural Alternatives for Weight Loss* (New York: William Morrow, 1996), viii.

5 "Obesity." *Nutrition Week* (July 28, 1995).

6 JoAnne E. Manson et al. "Body Weight and Mortality Among Women." *New England Journal of Medicine* 333:11 (1995), 677-685.

7 Jill Kelly, Ph.D. "Obesity: Nondiet Approaches for What's Eating Your Patients." *Alternative & Complementary Therapies* (October 1997), 326-332.

8 Lisa Grunwald. "Discovery: Do I look Fat to You? 28 Questions (and All the Answers) About Our National Obsession." *Life* (February 1, 1995),

58.

9 Ibid.

10 "America's Weight Problem Continues." Calorie Control Council press release (May 11, 1998). For more information, contact the Calorie Control Council at 404-252-3663.

11 Lisa Grunwald. "Discovery: Do I look Fat to You? 28 Questions (and All the Answers) About Our National Obsession." *Life* (February 1, 1995), 58.

12 National Institute of Diabetes and Digestive and Kidney Diseases. *Understanding Adult Obesity* NIH Publication No. 94-3680 (Washington: National Institutes of Health, 1998).

13 Susan McQuillan, M.S., R.D., with Edward Saltzman, M.D. *Complete Idiot's Guide to Losing Weight* (New York: Alpha Books, 1998), 29.

14 D. van Dale and W.H. Saris. "Repetitive Weight Loss and Weight Regain: Effects on Weight Reduction, Resting Metabolic Rate, and Lipolytic Activity Before and After Exercise and/or Diet Treatment." *American Journal of Clinical Nutrition* 49:3 (March 1989), 409-416.

Pain and Injuries

1 Office of Scientific and Health Reports, *National Institute of Neurological Disorders and Stroke. Chronic Pain—Hope Through Recovery* NIH Publication No. 90-2406 (Washington, DC: Dept. of Health and Human Services, Public Health Service, National Institutes of Health, 1989), 2.

2 R. O. Becker, *The Body Electric: Electro-Magnetism and the Foundation of Life* (New York: William Morrow, 1986). R. O. Becker, *Cross Currents* (Los Angeles: Jeremy P. Tarcher, 1990).

3 R. Sandyk, "The Influence of the Pineal Gland on Migraine and Cluster Headaches and Effects of Treatment with picoTesla Magnetic Fields." *International Journal of Neuroscience*

67:1-4 (November-December 1992), 145-171.

4 E. Riva Sanseverino, A. Vannini, and P. Castellacci. "Therapeutic Effects of Pulsed Magnetic Fields on Joint Diseases." *Panminerva Medica* 34:4 (October-December 1992), 187-196.

Respiratory Problems

1 R.M. Cherniack. *Respiration in Health and Disease* (Philadelphia: W.B. Saunders, 1983), 179.

2 E. Rubenstein and D.D. *Felderman, eds. Scientific American Medicine* (New York: Scientific American, 1982).

3 Ibid.

4 P. Austin. *Natural Remedies: A Manual* (Seale, AL: Yuchi Pines Institute, 1983).

5 *Physicians' Desk Reference* (Oradell, NJ: Medical Economics, 1990).

6 P. Austin. *Natural Remedies: A Manual* (Seale, AL: Yuchi Pines Institute, 1983).

7 G.A. Mozhaev and I.I. Tikhonovskii. "The Prevention and Treatment of Suppurative-Inflammatory Complications in the Bronchopulmonary System During Prolonged Artificial Ventilation." *Anesteziologiia i Reanimatologiia* 4 (July/August 1992), 47-51.

8 E. Cheraskin, M.D. *Vitamin C: Who Needs It* (Birmingham, AL: Arlington Press, 1993).

9 Ibid., 2.

10 Ibid., 9.

11 J.E. Pizzorno and M.T. Murray. *A Textbook of Natural Medicine* (Seattle, WA: John Bastyr College Publications, 1989).

Seizures

1 J.M. Faccini. "Fluoride-Induced Hyperplasia of the Parathyroid Glands." *Proceedings of the Royal Society of Medicine* 62 (1969), 241. L. Spira. "Fluorosis and the Parathyroid

Glands." *Journal of Hygiene* 42 (1942) 500-504. S.P.S. Teotia and M. Teotia. "Hyperactivity of the Parathyroid Glands in Endemic Osteofluorosis." *Fluoride* 5 (1972), 115-125.

Sleep Disorders

1 Arthur C. Guyton, M.D., and John E. Hall, Ph.D. *Textbook of Medical Physiology*, 9th Edition (Philadelphia: W.B. Saunders, 1996), 761.

2 Ibid.

3 H.J. Rinkel, T.G. Randolph, and M. Zeller. *Food Allergy* (Springfield, IL: Charles C. Thomas, 1950).

4 N. Ishida, M. Kaneko, and R. Allada. "Biological Clocks." *Proceedings of the National Academy of Sciences of the United States of America* 96:16 (August 3, 1996), 8819-8820.

5 Russel J. Reiter, Ph.D., and Jo Robinson. *Melatonin: Your Body's Natural Wonder Drug* (New York: Bantam Books, 1995), 17.

6 Russel J. Reiter, Ph.D., *Melatonin: Your Body's Natural Wonder Drug* (New York: Bantam Books, 1995). New York Academy of Sciences, "The Aging Clock," *Annals of New York Academy of Sciences*, Vol. 719, 1994. Ray Sahelian, M.D., *Melatonin: Nature's Sleeping Pill* (Marina Del Rey, CA: Be Happier Press, 1995). Walter Pierpaoli, M.D., Ph.D., Willaim Regelson, M.D., *The Melatonin Miracle* (New York: Simon & Schuster, 1995).

7 P. Semm. *Nature* 288 (December 11, 1980).

8 Robert O. Becker, M.D., *Cross Currents* (New York: G.P. Putnam's Sons, 1990).

9 A. Kahn et al. "Insomnia and Cow's Milk Allergy in Infants." *Pediatrics* 76:6 (December 1985), 880-884.

10 J. Martineau et al. "Vitamin B6, Magnesium, and Combined B6-Magnesium: Therapeutic Effects in Childhood Autism." *Biological Psychiatry* 20 (1985), 467-468.

11 M. Cohen and A. Bendich. "Safety of Pyridoxine: A Review of Human and Animal Studies." *Toxicology Letters* 34 (1986), 129-139.

12 L.M. Tierney, Jr., M.D. et al. *Current Medical Diagnosis & Treatment* (Norwalk, CT: Appleton & Lange, 1993).

13 S. Ayres and R. Mihan. "Leg Cramps and 'Restless Leg' Syndrome Responsive to Vitamin E (Tocopheral)." *California Medicine* 111:2 (1969), 87-91.

14 J. Penland. "Effects of Trace Element Nutrition on Sleep Patterns in Adult Women." *FASEB Journal* 2 (1988), A434.

15 J. Thom et al. "The Influence of Refined Carbohydrate on Urinary Calcium Excretion." *British Journal of Urology* 50 (1978), 459-464.

16 R.P. Heaney and C.M. Weaver. "Calcium Absorption From Kale." *American Journal of Clinical Nutrition* 51 (1990), 656-657.

17 B.P. Bourgoin et al. "Lead Content in 70 Brands of Dietary Calcium Supplements." *American Journal of Public Health* 83 (1993), 1155-1160.

18 J.A. Harvey et al. "Superior Calcium Absorption From Calcium Citrate Than Calcium Carbonate Using External Forearm Counting." *Journal of the American College of Nutrition* 9 (1990), 583-587.

19 C. Zhou et al. "Clinical Observation of Treatment of Hypertension with Calcium." *American Journal of Hypertension* 7 (1994), 363-367.

20 B.M. Altura. "Basic Biochemistry and Physiology of Magnesium: A Brief Review." *Magnesium and Trace Elements* 10 (1991), 167-171.

21 T. Bohmer et al. "Bioavailability of Oral Magnesium Supplementation in Female Students Evaluated From Elimination of Magnesium in 24-Hour Urine." *Magnesium and Trace Elements* 9 (1990), 272-278. L. Gullestad et al. "Oral Versus Intravenous Magnesium

Supplementation in Patients With Magnesium Deficiency." *Magnesium and Trace Element* 10 (1991), 11-16.

22 J.S. Lindberg et al. "Magnesium Bioavailability From Magnesium Citrate and Magnesium Oxide." *Journal of the American College of Nutrition* 9 (1990), 48-55.

23 Betty Kamen, Ph.D. *The Chromium Connection* (Novato, CA: Nutrition Encounter, 1992), 118.

24 W.W. Campbell and R.A. Anderson. "Effects of Aerobic Exercise and Training on the Trace Minerals Chromium, Copper, and Zinc." *Sports Medicine* 4 (1987), 9-18.

25 Jeffrey S. Bland, Ph.D. "Take Your Vitamins." *Delicious!* 8:7 (October 1992), 61.

26 James Perl, Ph.D. *Sleep Right in Five Nights* (New York: William Morrow/Quill, 1993), 236.

27 T.C. Birdsall. "5-Hydroxytryptophan: A Clinically Effective Serotonin Precursor." *Alternative Medicine Review* 3:4 (1998), 271-280.

28 R. Ursin. "The Effects of 5-Hydroxytryptophan and L-Tryptophan on Wakefulness and Sleep Patterns in the Cat." *Brain Research* 106:1 (1976), 105-115.

Women's Health Problems

1 R.F. Carey et al. "Effectiveness of Latex Condoms as a Barrier to Human Immunodeficiency Virus-Sized Particles Under Conditions of Simulated Use." *Sexually Transmitted Diseases* 19:4 (July/August 1992), 230-234.

2 G. Wilcox et al. "Oestrogenic Effects of Plant Foods in Postmenopausal Women." *British Medical Journal* 301:6757 (October 1990), 905-906.

3 H. Adlercreutz et al. "Dietary Phyto-Oestrogens and the Menopause in Japan." *The Lancet* 339:8803 (May 1992), 1233.

4 H. Adlercreutz et al. "Urinary Excretion of Lignans and Isoflavonoid Phytoestrogens in Japanese Men and Women Consuming a Traditional Japanese Diet." *American Journal of Clinical Nutrition* 54:6 (1991), 1093-1100.

5 S.M. Lark, M.D. *Dr. Susan Lark's The Menopause Self Help Book* (Berkeley, CA: Celestial Arts, 1990).

Index

diabetes and, 100
as heart disease factor, 128
obesity and, 102, 160
Food additives, 69, 89
Food families, 222
Foods
causes of reactions to, 216
elimination of, 166
irradiated, 69
mucus-producing, 72, 174
Foods, maladaptive reactions to, 86, 87, 122, 214–15
asthma and, 172
avoiding, 102
effects of, 151
as heart disease factor, 128
infections and, 138
lupus and, 141
MS and, 155–56
pain and, 166
as sleep disorder factor, 195
symptoms of, 124, 125
Four-Day Diversified Rotation Diet, 51, 214–21
for asthma, 173
for CFS, 92
for children, 87, 89
for food avoidance, 102
for food maladaptive reactions, 121
for heart conditions/disease, 130
for immune system strengthening, 86
for infections, 138
for inflammation, 139
as lifestyle, 153
for MS management, 155
for prostate problem prevention, 145
reintroduction of reactive foods, 166
Free radicals, 19, 20, 28, 32
effects of, 32, 115, 180
eliminating, 34–35, 115–16

heavy metals as, 70
overload, 73
Frequency, 18

Gaby, Alan, 117
Gangrene, 101
GAS (general adaptation syndrome), 98
Gastrointestinal problems, 119–25
Gauss, 17, 38
Gauss, Carl Friedrich, 17
Gauss rating, 38, 39
Gauss strength, 38, 39–40
General adaptation syndrome (GAS), 98
Genetics
in Alzheimer's disease, 55
in cancers, 74–75
in diabetes, 99
in seizures, 181
Genitourinary tract, male, 143
Geopathic stress, 65, 198
Gillespie, Larrian, 211–12
Glaucoma, 116
Gluten, 215
Gordon, Garry F., 59, 177
Grains, sprouted, 217

HBOT (hyperbaric oxygen therapy), 157–58
Head unit, 46
Headaches, 170, 204
Healing, 11
energy sources for, 79
negative magnetic fields for, 20, 24, 29–30, 164
Health problems, 11. See also Disease; Illness
Heart attack (myocardial infarction), 126, 127
Heart disease, 126–32
Hemorrhoids, 142
Herbicides, 66–67
Hernia, hiatal, 124
HGH. See Human growth hormone

for cancers, 76–78, 78–85
for cardiac pain, 132
for cerebral arteriosclerosis, 131
for CFS, 93, 95
for colds/sinusitis, 177
for colitis, 120–21
for constipation, 121–22
for depression, 97, 150
for detoxification, 58
devices for, 38
for diabetes, 105
for diverticulitis, 124
duration of, 81–82
for energy enhancement, 95
for environmental illness, 113
for eye disorders, 115–16
for food allergies, 122, 150–51
health conditions used for, 26–27
for heart conditions/disease, 127–28, 130, 132
for hiatal hernia, 124
history of, 21–25
for indigestion/nausea, 125
for infections, 93, 95, 135–37
for inflammation, 139–41
for irritable bowel syndrome, 125
for menstrual problems, 208–9
for mental disorders, 151–53
for MS, 156
noninvasive nature of, 26
for osteoporosis, 210
for overeating, 161
for pain relief, 165, 167–70
for parasites, 124
for prostate enlargement, 144
for seizures, 180–82
for sleep disorders, 198–99
strength of, 81–82
for symptom relief, 142
for weight loss, 161
for withdrawal, 161, 217
Magnetic deficiency, 19
Magnetic fields, 14, 15

external sources of, 19, 65
in human body, 17–19, 42
penetration, 38–39, 40, 41
retention of, 41–42
static, 15–16, 17
Magnetic resonance imaging (MRI), 20, 23
Magnetic shielding, 112
Magnetism, 15
Magnetoencephalography, 20
Magnetometer, 16
Magnets, 39
application of, 47–48
defined, 16
placement of, 38. See also name of condition to be treated
sizes, 43–45
types of, 38–40, 43–46
uses of, 14–15. See also Magnet therapy
Mats, 44, 46
Megavitamin therapy, 53
Melanoma, 77, 82–83
Melatonin, 24, 29, 35, 196–97
as antioxidant, 115, 116
in CFS, 96
defined, 34, 167
role in sleep, 80, 198–99
stimulation by negative fields, 116, 198, 199
suppression of, 141
Menopause, 209–10
Menstrual problems, 207–9
Mental disorders, 24, 147–53
Mercury, 56, 69–70, 109, 155
Metabolism
disordered, 54–55, 100
of fat, 161–62
fermentative, 32, 73, 75–76, 134
of microorganisms, 134, 135
Metal toxicity, 55–56, 56–57. See also Mercury
Metals, heavy, 67
Minerals, 201–3, 210
deficiencies, 53

solubility of, 55
Mini-blocks, 43, 45
Moles, 186–88
Mouth and lip cancers, 82
MRI (magnetic resonance imaging), 20, 23
Multiple sclerosis (MS), 154–58
Myocardial infarction, 126, 127

N-acetyl-cysteine, 118
NADH (nicotinamide adenine dinucleotide), 33
Nakagawa, Kyoichi, 19
Narcotics, 50, 214
Nash, J. Madeleine, 63
Nausea, 124–25
Negative fields, 14–15, 16, 29–36
  alkaline environment promotion by, 78, 115–16, 129, 214
  antibiotic effects, 133–34
  beneficial effects of, 19–20, 24, 26, 39, 164
  from body, 26, 29
  effects on brain, 181
  free radical elimination by, 115–16
  in healing, 20, 24, 29–30, 164
  melatonin production stimulation by, 116, 198, 199
  oxidoreductase enzyme stimulation by, 78, 112, 140, 153
  oxygenation by, 129, 135
Neodymium magnets, 16, 39, 45
Nerve blocks, 140, 163
Nerve deterioration, 101
Nerve interference fields, 70
Nervous system, 70, 112
Neurotransmitters, 195
Niacinamide, 103
Northrup, Christiane, 71
Nuclear radiation, 66
Nutrient absorption, 72, 94, 119
Nutritional deficiencies, 119
  in Alzheimer's disease, 56
  as cancer factor, 70–71, 86
  in CFS, 91–92

in constipation, 123
eyes and, 116, 117
in heart disease, 128
testing for, 94–95
Nutritional supplementation
  for addiction treatment, 53
  aging and, 117
  for Alzheimer's disease, 59
  for asthma, 173
  for bed-wetting, 88
  for boils, 184
  for bronchitis, 174
  for colds/sinusitis, 177
  for diabetes, 102–5
  for heart conditions/disease, 131
  for impotence, 145
  for infections, 138
  during menopause, 210
  for mental disorders, 153
  for pain relief, 166
  for seizure disorders, 182
  for sunburn, 189
  for warts/moles, 188

Oberg, Gary, 55
Obesity, 100, 102, 159–62
Oncogenes, 74
Osteoporosis, 210
Oxidation, 32, 34
Oxidation phosphorylation, 31, 75, 78
Oxidative Protection Screen, 95
Oxidoreductase enzymes, 19, 28, 32
  functioning of, 34–35, 153
  stimulation by negative fields, 78, 112, 140, 153
Oxyacids, 31, 32
Oxygen, 18, 75, 34
  anti-infectious properties, 135
  cancers and, 73–74, 75, 78
  deficiencies, 11, 73–74, 75, 164
  magnetizing, 58, 80, 84, 135, 175

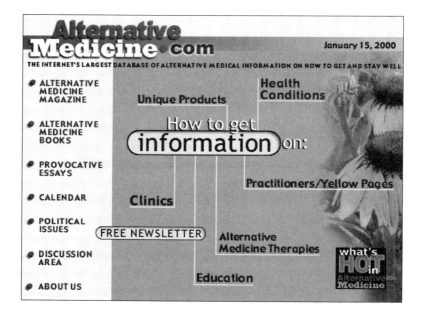

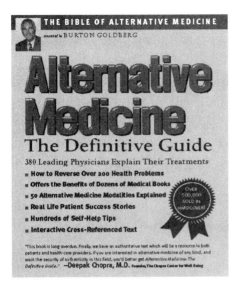

THE BIBLE OF ALTERNATIVE MEDICINE

edited by BURTON GOLDBERG

Alternative Medicine
The Definitive Guide

380 Leading Physicians Explain Their Treatments

- How to Reverse Over 200 Health Problems
- Offers the Benefits of Dozens of Medical Books
- 50 Alternative Medicine Modalities Explained
- Real Life Patient Success Stories
- Hundreds of Self-Help Tips
- Interactive Cross-Referenced Text

OVER 500,000 SOLD IN HARDCOVER!

"This book is long overdue. Finally, we have an authoritative text which will be a resource to both patients and health-care providers. If you are interested in alternative medicine of any kind, and want the security of authenticity in this field, you'd better get *Alternative Medicine: The Definitive Guide*." —Deepak Chopra, M.D. Founder, The Chopra Center for Well Being

Millions of people are searching for a better way to health—this is the book they're reaching for. *Alternative Medicine: The Definitive Guide* is an absolute must for anyone interested in the latest information on how to get healthy and stay that way.

At 1,100 pages, this encyclopedia puts all the schools of alternative medicine—50 different therapies—under one roof.

The *Guide* is packed with lifesaving information and alternative treatments from 380 of the world's leading alternative physicians. Our contributors give you the safest, most affordable, and most effective remedies for over 200 serious health conditions.

The *Guide* does something no other health book has ever done. It combines the best clinical information from doctors with the most practical self-help remedies all in a format that is easy-to-read, practical, and completely user-friendly.

The *Guide* gives you the knowledge you need today so you can make intelligent choices about the future of your health.

Now available in Spanish

To order, call 800-333-HEAL or visit www.alternativemedicine.com.
You can also find our books at your local health food store or bookstore.

national book network

BOOKS
your health
depends on

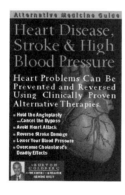

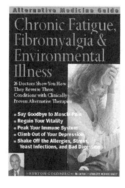

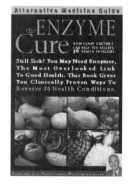

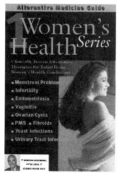

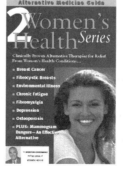

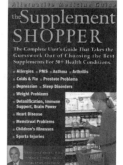

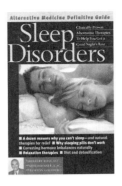
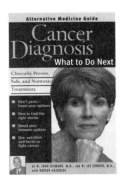
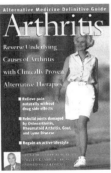
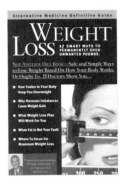

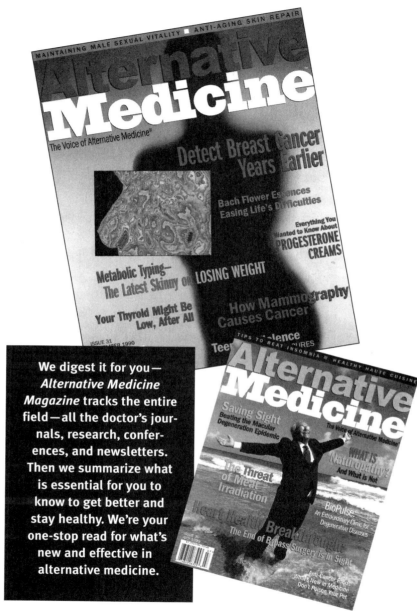

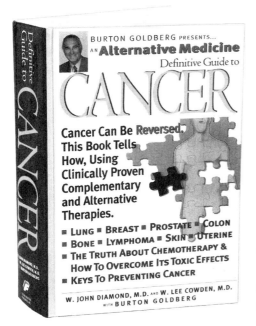

CURE YOUR HEADACHES...USING NATURAL THERAPIES

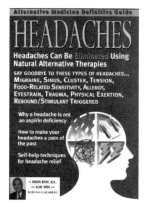

If you suffer from headaches, this book could change your life. It is entirely possible that with this invaluable practical information, you may well put headaches behind you as something you once suffered from, but no more.

Robert Milne, M.D., and Blake More expertly guide you through the root causes and multiple treatment options for 11 major types of headaches.

We have made every effort possible to make this book practical and user-friendly for you. For a quick reference to headache types, symptoms, treatment options, use our Master Symptom Chart. If you suffer from tension headaches, turn directly to Chapter 6; if migraines are your millstone, see Chapter 7; and if you're not sure what type of headache you have, study the symptoms list in the Master Symptom Chart until you find the clinical term that best matches your condition.

No matter what kind of headache you used to have, after reading this book your head may never pain you again.

Trade paper ■ ISBN 1-887299-18-1 ■ 6" x 9" ■ 525 pages

To order, call 800-333-HEAL or visit www.alternativemedicine.com. You can also find our books at your local health food store or bookstore.

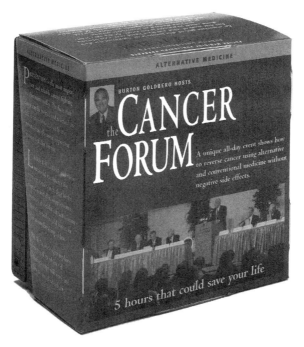

The Cancer Forum—five hours of lifesaving information from leading alternative medicine physicians who show you how to reverse cancer using alternative and conventional medicine without negative side effects.

Prevention is the most important and reliable cancer-fighting tool that exists today. The fact that cancer can be treated and reversed and that it can be detected early and prevented are the most significant messages of this forum.

Learn the latest proven, safe, nontoxic, and successful treatments for reversing cancer, including herbs, nutrition and diet, supplements, enzymes, glandular extracts, homeopathic remedies, and more, in this groundbreaking video.

TO ORDER, CALL 800-333-HEAL

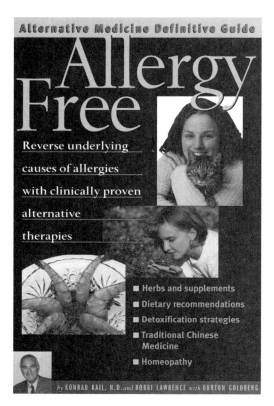

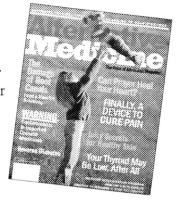

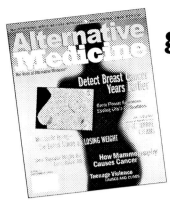

give yourself
the GIFT
of HEALTH
subscribe today!

www.alternativemedicine.com